Jewish Pastoral Insights On Senior Residential Care

Flourishing In The Later Years

Rabbi James R. Michaels
Rabbi Cary Kozberg

D1251189

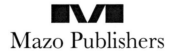

Mazo Publishers

Flourishing In The Later Years

ISBN: 978-1-936778-93-5

Second Edition

Published by:
Mazo Publishers
Jacksonville, Florida
Tel: 1-815-301-3559

Email: mazopublishers@gmail.com
Website: www.mazopublishers.com

About The Front Cover Image:
"The Tree of Life," created by the residents and staff of
Lieberman Center in Skokie, Illinois, and currently displayed in
the synagogue at Lieberman.

For Karen

And for Sheryl

Thanks for being present!

CONTENTS

The Editors

Rabbi James R. Michaels, D. Min, BCC, is the Director of Pastoral Care at the Charles E. Smith Life Communities, formerly called the Hebrew Home of Greater Washington, in Rockville, MD. Since assuming this position in 2003, he has been an integral part of the culture change process, helping to develop the institution's value statement and to improve end-of-life pastoral care.

Before moving to Rockville, he served congregations and health-care facilities in Whitestone, NY, Wilkes-Barre, PA, and Flint, MI. He is also a CPE Diplomate Supervisor, teaching chaplaincy skills to clergy, seminarians, and laity. Rabbi Michaels is Professor of Jewish Studies at the Graduate Theological Foundation, Mishawaka, IN. He has published numerous articles in professional and scholarly journals, both in print and on-line.

Rabbi Cary Kozberg, BCC, is the Director of Religious Life at Wexner Heritage Village in Columbus, Ohio, where he has created and developed religious and spiritual programs for both Jewish and non-Jewish residents, their families and WHV staff.

Before assuming his position in 1989, he served two congregations and was the Hillel Director at the University of Texas in Austin. Rabbi Kozberg is a Past Chair of the Forum on Religion Spirituality and Aging and has written and presented extensively on the topic of spirituality and aging. Among his many publications is *Honoring Broken Tablets: A Jewish Approach to Dementia* (Jewish Lights Publishing).

Preface

James R. Michaels and Cary Kozberg

After my second stroke, my family and I had to make some decisions. We could have gotten someone to come in every day or every other day to help me, so that I could have continued to live in my own home. But since I can't drive any more, and most of my friends (those who are still around) can't drive either, I would have been "independent" but very isolated. And who wants to sit around the house all day by themselves?

In some ways, moving to a nursing home was not such a hard decision. I know most people don't even like to think about spending the rest of their days in a nursing home. But I believe it's all in how you approach it. I told my daughter that since I won't have to worry about a lot of things that now are concerns – like preparing meals, doing laundry – I can concentrate on creating a life that will have real quality; doing the kinds of activities that I like – stimulating my body and my brain, being with people I like – all in an environment that is Jewish and familiar.

Miriam K

The Psalmist writes, "Still in old age, they bring forth fruit."[1] It has always been assumed that the verse refers idealistically to the rewards reaped in later years by the righteous for the good works of their younger years. However, many senior citizens might question whether length of years is a reward for anything. Burdened with aches and illnesses, and having experienced significant losses, those in the so-called golden years might prefer to have less of the psalm's promised reward. If asked, almost all seniors will say they don't want their last home to be a nursing home. But then there are people like Miriam, who resonate with the psalm's words and spirit, and believe that their lives can be rich and productive in old age, even in a skilled nursing facility.

---

1   Psalm 92.15.

As chaplains in senior residential care facilities, we view our institutions as places of opportunity, not just for people like Miriam, but for all our residents, regardless of their medical conditions. Over the years we have observed our residents discover that they still have the potential to live, love, and create. Far from being "the last stop" on life's journey, senior residential care facilities can empower and energize individuals in ways they or their families would not have envisioned.

Pastoral care can help all persons of faith to realize this potential, and certainly those who are Jewish. Some residents in senior residential care bring a life-long history of Jewish religious observance which they seek to replicate in their new environment. Others may have been minimally observant, but find personal satisfaction in their twilight years by connecting with their religious heritage, as they participate in services and Jewish cultural programs. Still others may not be committed to religious observance at all, but find comfort in the Jewish cultural ambience created by the availability of kosher food and religious services.

Needless to say, seniors in senior residential care confront a variety of health care issues. Cognizant of these problems, Jewish chaplains who serve in such settings have the ability to present the traditions and teachings of Judaism in innovative ways which, again, can enrich the lives of their residents. For example, though Jewish residents with Alzheimer's Disease may not recognize and enjoy new liturgical music (currently very popular in synagogues), they still may respond to melodies and songs which are "old standards" from their younger days. For those residents who may not be comfortable spending long periods of time away from their rooms, technology offers various ways of bringing religious services to them. With short-term memory loss so prevalent among nursing home residents, it is often difficult for this cohort to build a knowledge base of new information. In such circumstances, the traditional role of rabbi-as-teacher can evolve to one of affirming listener, offering a simple "ministry of presence".

We decided to write this book because of the relatively small body of literature dealing with Jewish pastoral care, especially on the subject of long-term care. Over the years, articles have appeared in various journals of pastoral care, social work, and Jewish communal service.[2]

---

2   Articles can be found in *Journal of Pastoral Care, Journal on Jewish Aging, Jewish Spiritual Care,* among others. Melvin A. Kimble, Susan A.

The first book to address the subject was Rabbi Dayle Friedman's *Jewish Pastoral Care*; it contains several articles on long-term care.[3] Rabbi Jack Bloom's *Jewish Relational Care A to Z*,[4] also addresses issues which are germane to the subject of senior care.

In 2008, Rabbi Friedman published *Jewish Visions for Aging*.[5] It is invaluable for the guidance it provides for families and caregivers, as well as the lists of resources at the end of each chapter. Its value will grow in the future, as senior care becomes less institutional and more home-based. Although several chapters are devoted to long-term pastoral care, the work of chaplains is addressed in only a few chapters.

As we set out to write this book, we realized there are many aspects of Jewish pastoral care in senior residential settings. As with all aspects of health care chaplaincy, many deal with clinical issues affecting patient-care. Unlike our colleagues in acute care chaplaincy, Jewish long-term care chaplains spend significant amounts of time creating religious and cultural programs to nurture the spirits and enrich the lives of our residents. And because of the wide range of emotional and spiritual needs of residents in long-term care, these programs always require new and creative approaches.

With this in mind, we have divided this volume into three parts:

Clinical issues: How Jewish pastoral care makes a direct impact on the lives of the seniors in residential care. Our contributors address issues affecting not just individual residents, but also their families, caregivers, and the larger community.

Pastoral programming: How those engaged in Jewish pastoral care in senior residential care facilities enhance resident care through various programmatic innovations. We've included chapters about Torah study, prayer, Israel, and bereavement – topics which fit into the purview of Jewish pastoral care. There are also chapters which demonstrate how Jewish chaplains can interface with the work of creative arts and rehabilitative therapy.

What the future will bring: As the nature of senior residential

---

McFadden, *et al.* have published *Aging, Spirituality, and Religion,* a series of anthologies which present many issues of pastoral care for seniors, although not from an exclusively Jewish perspective.

3   Jewish Lights Publishing, First edition, 2001; second edition, 2005.

4   Haworth Press, 2006.

5   Jewish Lights Publishing.

care in this country rapidly changes, Jewish nursing homes and social agencies serving the elderly will join their non-Jewish sister organizations in seeking ways to respond. Regulatory changes, as well as evolving insurance payment issues will create new economic realities, as well as consequences for the emotional and spiritual well-being of residents and staff. We present two chapters which address these possibilities.

As thorough as we have tried to be in this survey, we do not presume that it is exhaustive, or that we have included every aspect or innovation in the field. Indeed, we understand that many chaplains' creative work has not come to our attention. We salute their efforts and anticipate that future books and articles will be written that will include their contributions to the field.

When we began collecting articles, we realized we wanted to appeal to several different audiences:

- Jewish chaplains already working in the field, seeking ideas to enhance their work.
- Administrators in Jewish senior residential care settings, considering how to improve service to their residents.
- Administrators and chaplains in non-Jewish facilities, looking to provide spiritual care for Jewish residents.
- Those who work in the direct-care disciplines – nursing, social work, recreational therapy – who often collaborate with Jewish chaplains.
- Lay people, concerned about making choices for their aging relatives.

As a result, we requested articles which are not necessarily "scholarly" in approach. At the same time, we welcomed annotations and bibliographies. We encouraged contributors to write from their own experiences. Many articles reflect their authors' passion built of successes or frustrations. Wherever possible, we have stayed away from Jewish and professional jargon. When Hebrew, Yiddish and Jewish terms are used, they have been translated or explained in the text. Of course, we welcome feedback and suggestions from those who will read this book.

Psalm 119:99 states, "I have learned much from all my teachers." This could be the watchword of the work of chaplaincy, which is to listen and learn from those we serve. Thus we dedicate this book to our teachers:

- Our CPE supervisors, who gave us the initial training to pursue our dreams of chaplaincy.
- Senior care professionals who we believe toil "the vineyards of the Lord", and have taught us the sacred minutiae of patient care.
- Our residents – those still with us and those who have passed on – who have taught us about their lives, fears, and joys.

Since they are too numerous to mention, we trust our teachers will recognize who they are and share in the pride we feel in this book.

January, 2009
Tevet, 5769

Preface To The Second Edition

Since we published the first edition, we have been gratified by the favorable response we've received from readers throughout the United States and around the world. We felt justified for having undertaken the project, and feel we have succeeded in making a contribution to the field of geriatric pastoral care.

Although only two years have passed since the publication of our first edition, several significant events have transpired affecting the field of aging services, and the work of chaplains in senior residential settings:

- The emergence of the "Culture Change" movement in senior residential care, aiming to alter elder care from a hospital-based model to one which stresses the individuality of each resident. Thus we have changed the term "long-term care" to "senior residential care," stressing the continuum of care, depending on each individual's specific needs.
- The passage of the Patient Protection and Affordable Care Act (i.e. health care reform) in 2010. This law contains provisions which will impact on the nursing home industry, and may change the ways seniors receive care in the future.
- The opening of the first Jewish "Green House" residences in Dedham, MA. This new model of skilled nursing care has been hailed as a great step forward; the Jewish pastoral response to this new model of care will be instructive for other facilities in the future.
- The increasing use of technology to improve the lives of those in residential care.

And, of course, we have learned of innovations by our colleagues and wanted to include them in this volume.

We are grateful to all of our contributors, as well to those who have encouraged us to bring this second edition to fruition.

Naturally, we want to acknowledge the love and support of our families who have stood by us throughout our careers: Karen Markowitz Michaels; Marnin and Melissa, Aaron and Limor, Dania and Stu, Aliza and Gal, Etzion and Danielle; Julia, Lauren, Maya, Noa, Brody, Alon, Shai and Chase.

Sheryl Kozberg; Zak, Shoshi, Ben and Adina, and Jake; Marcy Kozberg and Bernard Kozberg, of blessed memory, and Ellen Kozberg.

Finally we want once again to acknowledge and thank our fellow chaplains. Let us go from strength to strength as we seek to serve our patients and, in the process do the will of, and bring glory to, our Creator.

Jim Michaels
Cary Kozberg
November 2011
Heshvan 5772

Introduction

Dr. Stephen Sapp

An Incredible Adventure

A popular item that has made the Internet rounds regularly since its original appearance in *The Onion*[1], carries the alarming headline, "World Death Rate Holding Steady At 100 Percent." The article goes on to assert that death "has long been considered humanity's number one health concern" and is "responsible for 100 percent of all recorded fatalities worldwide," noting somberly that "the condition has no cure." One "expert" is quoted as observing that "it is beginning to seem possible that birth – as well as the subsequent life cycle that follows it – may be a serious safety risk for all those involved."

Indeed it is! Although intended as a parody, this article accurately conveys a fundamental truth – perhaps *the* fundamental truth – about human existence, and significantly this truth is one of the few points of agreement among all the world's religions: Human beings are mortal, and every one of us will experience death, the end of each person's existence on this planet. This incontrovertible (and inescapable!) fact leads to – or perhaps stems from – what is arguably the beginning and ending points for religion, namely, that *this* earthly existence is not what human life is all about. Different religions present various reasons for this situation; they offer vastly differing visions of what follows death; and they suggest diverse ways in which one should live one's life. But they agree – as *The Onion*'s spoof reminds us – that we all *will* die.

I am more vividly aware of this fact at this moment in my life than I have ever been. I am writing this exactly four weeks after my 96-year-old father died from chronic lymphocytic leukemia and as my 94-year-old mother is in the hospital for congestive heart failure and

---

1   Issue 31.02, January 22, 1997.

viral pneumonia. I recognize that I am very blessed to have been able to come within months of my 65th birthday (the long-accepted age for being "old" in our country) with both parents still alive and in relatively sound health until very recently. But some time soon I too will join the majority among my age group (and even younger) who are orphans. Although I have worked in the field of gerontology for almost three decades, have been an ordained Presbyterian minister for yet another before that, and regularly teach university-level courses in death and dying and various aspects of biomedical ethics, I cannot shake the feeling that my life is taking a new and dramatic direction.

So where are these personal musings leading us in terms of the theme of this book? The above-mentioned article from *The Onion* provides the starting-point to answer that question in the following statement: "Many are suggesting that the high mortality rate represents a massive failure on the part of the planet's health care workers." And a "concerned parent" is quoted as saying, "The inability of doctors and scientists to adequately address this issue of death is nothing less than a scandal." Although intended as satire, both of those statements are close enough to reflecting the real attitude of many contemporary Americans to give one pause: A large number of people today *do* hope fervently – perhaps even *expect* – that modern scientific techno-medicine will find a cure for aging and death, and an "anti-aging movement" is flourishing as its advocates work diligently to make that hope a reality.

Thoughts such as these often call to my mind the Cheshire cat's reply to Alice's inquiry, "Would you please tell me which way I ought to go from here?" That famous cat, doubtlessly grinning, said, "That depends on where you want to get to." I think we need to give a great deal more thought than is currently being given to the critical question of what constitutes the destination that I assume we all want to reach (and what it will take to reach it): the magnificent biblical ideal of "a good old age" – the best image I can think of to describe quality (or "successful," or "healthy") aging.

If we are to achieve that goal, however, it obviously matters a great deal where our starting point is. Unfortunately, as *The Onion* article suggests, the dominant cultural response to aging in the United States today is that it is an affront to our innate right to "life, liberty, and the pursuit of happiness" and should be eliminated. Further, growing old is increasingly perceived not as the natural course of human (and all other) life but rather a challenge for medicine to conquer – an illness, a disease, that somehow violates the natural order and should be fought at all costs. Not surprisingly, then, adherents of this approach maintain that if we only place our faith in modern medical science, it will find a way to save us from getting old (and the obvious companion of aging, death). As with any idol, however – whether it be a golden calf at the foot of Mt. Sinai or a more modern one like anti-aging medicine – ultimately it will fail to provide us with what we most need as we inevitably age and are forced to confront our own deaths.

Why can scientific medicine not give us what we need for our quest to reach a "good old age"? The answer is simple: because our basic view of aging and death, and thus of people who are old and dying, is not based on science and facts, though obviously certain facts are relevant. Questions regarding aging and death – what it *means* to grow old and die and how one should relate to people who are old – are not scientific questions at all, but rather *theological/philosophical* questions; they are questions of *value* which science acknowledges is not its realm. Despite our indisputable nature as biological organisms, our species *homo sapiens* is not merely a biological entity, nothing more than creatures of the earth that will ultimately return to it (though we must never lose sight of the reality of that aspect of our nature). Although we definitely need food, shelter, and health care to live fulfilling lives, our admittedly *earthen* bodies are animated by the very breath of the Divine. Thus, we are also *spiritual* creatures who need love, community, and meaning at least as much.

Recalling the lyrics of that memorable Beatles song, "Will you still need me, will you still feed me, when I'm 64?", even if we update for our expanded life span today, of course it will be important that someone *feed* us when we are 84 or even 94, but it may be even more important that someone *need* us because, ultimately, whatever meaning life will hold for us at that age will not come from the material things that are so central to us when we are younger. That is a teaching of virtually all the world's religions and it is corroborated by the experience of life. In short, the questions of what growing older means and how one should respond to it, both with regard to oneself and others, go beyond any scientific, factual analysis or discussion to a fundamental understanding of the nature and purpose of human life itself. Therefore the discovery of a "good old age" (though certainly enhanced by good health) ultimately lies in the realm of a person's values and his/her understanding of human existence – what might be called broadly the "spiritual" realm.[2]

So when contemporary scientific biomedicine reaches the end of its capabilities to extend and enhance life, impressive as those achievements have been and will continue to be, what is left for elders and those charged with their care? Where can we turn to find some guidance in challenging the dominant values of our society that seem to be taking us to a place where meaning and hope are increasingly hard for us to find and/or hold onto as we age? Religion (or spirituality if one prefers a more contemporary approach) offers precisely what science cannot, that "Something More" that is desperately needed as one confronts one's mortality face-on. The painfully difficult existential question that we contemporary Americans face – "What meaning, what purpose is there to living if I just have to get old and die?" – is precisely the question which this book sets out to answer.

Focusing on the clinical and programmatic aspects of pastoral care in Jewish senior residential facilities, this book demonstrates that religion (Judaism, specifically, but all religious traditions as well) can provide answers to the existential questions associated with aging. Indeed, those who work in these facilities hear residents and their families, and other staff, asking such questions, perhaps daily, and in different ways. The various modalities of pastoral care presented in this book will hopefully provide some measure of succor and encouragement.

Several years ago I had the privilege of hosting the distinguished German Protestant Christian theologian Jürgen Moltmann for three days in Miami.[3] As part of his visit, I was able to interview him for an

2   I would note that by emphasizing the importance of spiritual concerns in the lives of older people, I certainly do not mean to downplay the importance or necessity of the best possible scientific research into aging or the central role that biological, social, and cultural factors play in producing a quality old age. I am merely saying that an approach that never goes beyond these factors, that never recognizes the central importance of this spiritual realm and the issues coming forth from it, is necessarily incomplete because, for all its successes and contributions, it can never reveal to us the meaning of our lives and our deaths.

3   Although a prolific thinker and writer (he recently completed a six-volume *magnum opus* called *Systematic Contributions to Theology*), Professor Moltmann is undoubtedly best known in the United States for a book that appeared in English in 1967 as *The Theology of Hope: On the Ground and the Implications of a Christian Eschatology* (New York: Harper and Row, 1967).

hour about his own aging (he had just turned 73) and the relationship between his theology and growing older. I asked him if *I* could still relate to God if *I* lost my higher mental functions, as for example in the case of dementia. After a moment of reflection, he replied, "*You* may not be able to relate to God, but *God* can still be in relationship with you. It's not just your relationship to God but also God's relationship to you, and that's the more important one." This notion is extremely potent and important in helping us to affirm that there is an ongoing meaning to living, amid even the worst degenerative changes that sometimes accompany aging. Certainly the good professor's words should serve as a prophetic source of both resistance and hope in the face of our society's apparent determination to devalue people whose control of their will and understanding may be slipping away as they age.

Certainly those who affirm the God of Abraham can find great comfort in this view of God's relationship to human beings, even as we experience the unavoidable changes of life: Whether we are personally facing the losses and inevitable outcome of aging, or we are a family member, friend, or professional facing the prospect of caring for someone throughout that process, *God never forgets* us, and in that affirmation lies genuine hope. It is out of this affirmation that Professor Moltmann describes his own experience of aging: "*(Aging) has remained for me until today an incredible adventure, a voyage of discovery into a country that is unknown to me, and a departure without the safety of a return. (Aging) is for me an open, inviting way with many surprises.*"

I commend the editors and authors of this second edition of *Flourishing In The Later Years: Jewish Pastoral Insights On Senior Residential Care* for recognizing the indispensable nature of the spiritual dimension of aging and for providing a resource that is both practical and seriously grounded in Judaism, one of the oldest and greatest religious traditions of humankind. Although appropriately focused on that tradition, this book will be of value and considerable assistance to those of any spiritual background who interact with elders and to all of us as we continue along the "incredible adventure" of our own aging, making our own "voyage of discovery" into that unknown country.

Part One – Clinical Issues

Chapter 1

You Shall Be Holy: The Roles Of The Jewish Chaplain In Senior Residential Care Settings[1]

Rabbi Cary Kozberg

It can be difficult to hold someone's attention after you mention that you work in a nursing home, or a rehabilitations hospital (unless you can tell a triumphant story of recovery), or a residential facility for persons with disabilities. Perhaps this is because human beings prefer to avoid thinking about the circumstances that might land them in long-term care. Perhaps it's because Americans prefer to avoid thinking about how to provide for the long-term care of some of society's most vulnerable members.[2]

As one who has worked as a chaplain in senior residential care facilities (SRCs) for over twenty years, I have been an eyewitness to the truth of these words almost on a daily basis. Hardly a week goes by that I am not asked, "How do you do what you do?" Hardly a day goes by that I don't see that look of visible discomfort, anxiety and even fear on the faces of visitors walking through our doors. Sometimes I wonder: who can fault them? How can a person not help feeling disoriented and anxious in the presence of so many who have lost youthfulness, beauty, vitality, cognition, and may be left feeling only despair and sorrow? Why *wouldn't* visitors naturally feel a sense of dread, and an immediate desire to turn heel and flee?

In our culture, agencies that serve and house the very frail and disabled are places that are mostly ignored (at best) or avoided (at

---

1   This chapter is dedicated to the memory of my mother Marcy Kozberg z"l, who was unmindful of how much sanctity she created.

2   Nancy Berlinger *Plainviews*, Vol 5, No. 8.

worst) because they are the very antithesis of what our culture is about: youthfulness, beauty, vitality, productivity, and most of all, independence. Through media coverage, the public's knowledge/awareness of life in SRCs usually centers on resident abuse, with hardly a mention of the countless acts of love and caring that occur every day.

Yet, while it may be accurate to say that the aforementioned attributes are indeed those which our culture cherishes (idolizes?), it is the presence or absence of those acts of love and caring that should give a truer perspective of our culture. As Rabbi Abraham J. Heschel noted:

> ...*the true standard by which to gauge a culture is the extent to which reverence, compassion and justice are to be found in the daily lives of a whole people, not only in the acts of isolated individuals.* Culture is a style of living compatible with the grandeur of being human *(italics his)*. *A test of a people is how it behaves toward the old.*[3]

That SRCs in general (and nursing homes in particular) are often considered places to be avoided and shunned is an attitude confirmed by the often-expressed words of older parents to their adult children: "Promise me you'll never put me in one of *those* places." Given these widely held feelings in our culture, it is easy to see why Rabbi Heschel's observation is still as true today as it was a half-century ago: "the care for the old is regarded as an act of charity rather than as a supreme privilege."[4]

Indeed, sometimes caring for the elderly *is* an act of charity. And sometimes it makes for a profitable business. Neither necessarily detracts from the need or the importance. Whether their motives are altruistic, economic, or a bit of both, institutions that provide residential senior care know that a certain standard of excellence and dedication is desired and expected by residents, families, communities, and even the government.

Facilities that strive to be "successful" are usually dedicated to providing care and service which reflect a commitment to "excellence,"

---

3   Abraham J. Heschel "To Grow in Wisdom" *The Insecurity of Freedom,* New York: Schocken, 1972, p. 72. This paper was first presented at the 1961 White House Conference on Aging.

4   Ibid., p.70.

"resident-centered quality of life," "a high standard of professionalism," along with a commitment to efficiency and cost-effectiveness.[5] Yet, as organizations that care for the elderly strive to meet these goals in an ever more challenging economic and political environment, caring for the frail elderly will be more an economic challenge and less an act of charity, much less a privilege.

Still, for many who work directly with residents of SRCs – those who provide or witness countless gestures of love and compassion every day – it remains more of a privilege than an act of charity. Indeed, some staff members with whom I've worked have described their roles as "deputized shepherds" – being present with folks as they sojourn in the "Valley of the Shadow", and helping to prepare them to pass from this life to the next. Such individuals tend to see their work as *sacred.*

The words "sacred" and "holy" are religious words; they are not usually heard in secular settings such as board rooms, clinics, or other business venues. But in places that serve and house the frail elderly, particularly those under "faith-based" auspices, they are adjectives that are not only appropriate, but arguably necessary: they best describe what "faith-based" senior residential care should strive to be. Yes, it is expected that "good" care will be both compassionate and cost-efficient. But in my experience, those agencies that provide the best care are most successful because they *consciously* are motivated by "a higher purpose". Although not necessarily articulated in mission statements or other venues, there is an embedded belief in their organizational culture that through the care they give, they are bringing God's presence into places which our culture often dismisses as "God-forsaken."

Of course, interpreting their missions/objectives in this way flows from a certain theological perspective – namely promoting a sense of the holy and sacred *(kedushah)*. From a specifically *Jewish* perspective, increasing holiness and sanctity in the world is an expectation of covenantal responsibility that is incumbent on the Jewish community, both collectively and individually: "You shall be holy, for I the Lord your

---

5   Two initiatives for promoting better quality in long-term care have been the government-sponsored the Nursing Home Quality Initiative, and Quality First, the counterpart initiative of AAHSA (now Leading Age), the American Health Care Association and the Alliance for Quality Nursing Home Care. Both programs have also led to other initiatives like Advancing Excellence in America's Nursing Homes and recent culture change advancements, exemplified by the Pioneer Network and the Eden Alternative.

God am holy."[6] Notably, this general commandment is followed several verses on by a specific one focusing the needs of the elderly.[7]

From this biblical mandate comes the reason and necessity for Jewish pastoral care, particularly in senior residential care settings where Jewish people live. While it is hoped that every staff member who works in an SRC is motivated by this "higher purpose", the overall goal of Jewish pastoral care is to affirm *kedushah*/sanctity within these settings – to help others recognize it, and to seek its actualization in all aspects of a facility's life and culture.

To be sure, a Jewish understanding of promoting and actualizing *kedushah*/sanctity is not limited to the familiar realms of ritual, ceremony, or sacred learning, but includes the realm of ethical behavior as well.[8] Thus, from a Jewish perspective, fostering *kedushah*/sanctity in senior residential care settings ideally focuses on two areas:

- Promoting those actions/behaviors that are usually thought of as "religious" – worship, Sabbath and holiday observances, dietary rules (*kashrut*), Torah study, and religious education.
- Seeking to insure that ethical and interpersonal relations – among residents and families, between the facility and residents/families, between the administration and staff, and among staff members themselves – also reflect this sacred commitment.

The "4 Ps"

As the "go-to" person for matters Jewish, the Jewish chaplain in an SRC is the *mara d'atra*, the on-site religious authority. In this capacity, he/she assumes four distinct roles – the *priestly*, the *pastoral*, the *pedagogic*, and the *prophetic*.

The "Priestly" Role

As individuals age and cope with the changes and losses that accompany growing older, the need to re-order one's life becomes more important. Indeed, one of the most critical tasks for the elderly person is

---

6   Leviticus 19:2.

7   Leviticus 19:32.

8   Many of the ethical commandments are found in Leviticus 19, which is also referred to as "The Holiness Code".

to retain a sense of identity, a "sense of sameness," as they face physical decline and the losses that accompany advanced age.[9] This re-ordering of a person's life includes being able to "let go" of youth, beauty, and status, while working to cultivate a self whose worth is measured in things closer to the heart.

Religion's role in helping to sustain a person's spiritual self can be significant here. Religious teachings, symbols, and rituals play an important part in assuring an elderly person that life will continue to hold meaning and that there will be continuity between past and present.[10] As Rabbi Heschel again put it so eloquently:

> *Upon reaching the summit of his years, man discovers that entertainment is no substitute of celebration … And he also knows that, in all his deeds, man's chief task is to sanctify time.*[11]

Like chaplains of other faiths, the priestly role of Jewish chaplains in SRCs is to help residents "celebrate" and sanctify time. Like their non-Jewish colleagues, they facilitate regular daily or weekly worship, special holiday services and other religious ceremonies for the various Jewish holidays throughout the year (e.g. Passover Seders, Hanukah candle-lighting, etc.). Within this priestly role, they help Jewish residents continue to mark Jewish sacred times, both happy and sad, and thus help them to connect both with God and with the larger community of faith through its sacred liturgy.[12]

---

9   Bernice Neugarten, quoted in *Enabling the Elderly: Religious Institutions With the Community Service System* by Sheldon Tobin, James, W. Ellor, and Susan M. Anderson Ray 1986, SUNY Press, p. 4.

10   Cf. Lea Pardue's study on the spiritual needs of frail elderly residents in long-term care settings in *The Journal of Religious Gerontology*, Vol. 8 (1), 1991. One of her findings was that although attendance at formal worship services may decrease as a person ages, personal belief and practice may grow stronger.

11   Heschel, ibid., p. 74 and p. 82. The challenge of sanctifying time that is often experienced by residents as "routinized" and empty is amply addressed by Rabbi Dayle Friedman in her article "Spiritual Challenges of Nursing Home Life" in *Aging, Spirituality and Religion*, edited by M. Kimble, S. McFadden, J. Ellor and J. Seeber, 1995, Fortress Press, pp. 362-373.

12   Although the adjective "*priestly*" is employed here when referring to a chaplain's liturgical responsibilities, the Jewish community has not had a functioning priestly class whose liturgical responsibilities were exclusive, since

In this capacity, Jewish chaplains also play a crucial role in helping residents and their families mark important milestones on life's journey, especially when the journey is coming to an end. In these moments, they may be called upon to offer prayers at the bedsides of sick or dying residents, or to officiate at their funerals. While these duties always have the potential to lapse into mere perfunctory rituals, the sensitive chaplain guards against this by remembering and reflecting on his/her priestly sacred responsibility in the moment. Amid the feelings of anxiety, and sorrow felt by others, he/she is the symbol of hope, strength and certainty, representing God's infinite caring, and the familial connection between the resident (and family) and the larger faith community of Israel. (See The "Pastoral" Role.)

I would add that there are two rituals which have been added to the religious/spiritual program of some SRCs that acknowledge both the sanctity and the challenges of specific "moments of transition" in the lives of residents, and have been shown to have tremendous positive emotional and spiritual impact on them and their families. The first is a *ceremony of welcoming*, conducted for a resident (and his/her family) when he/she first moves into an SRC. Because such a move marks a major life transition in the lives of the resident and his/

---

biblical times. On the contrary, unlike other faith communities which require that only ordained clergy perform liturgical functions, Jewish tradition since the first century CE has required only that a prayer leader have an aesthetically-pleasing voice, a working knowledge of the liturgy itself, and be personally pious. Ordination and/or other evidence of advanced theological knowledge are not requirements, which is one reason that ordination is not a requirement to serve as a Jewish chaplain (but sufficient clinical training is!). However, as the liturgical "representative" of the people to God, the worship leader – whether ordained or layperson – does serve in a "priestly" capacity, as does his/her counterpart in other cultures.

Given the fact that a layperson can serve in this role, the question might be asked: is having a trained chaplain on staff a necessity? In an era of shrinking budgets, the consideration of utilizing lay volunteers or clergy from local synagogues instead of trained chaplains is always present. However, many administrators and CEO's of Jewish-sponsored SRCs believe that "the mission of their facilities is to serve the *entire* Jewish community" (Warren Slavin, CEO of the Charles E. Smith Life Communities in Rockville, MD). Since there are a wide variety of religious practices in the community, it is necessary to have a professionally-trained chaplain who will respect and respond to the varying needs across the population of an SRC.

her family, it is often accompanied by a myriad of thoughts and feelings around the changes that separation and loss bring. Acknowledging the transition in a formal, liturgical way treats it as a rite of passage, like birth, adolescence, marriage, parenthood and death. Like other rites of passage, a ceremony of welcoming can help give meaning to the changes in role and status that are experienced. It can clarify that a new stage of life has begun, while facilitating closure of the previous stage. In these ways, it means to accomplish an additional purpose – it can offer hope.[13]

The second ritual is a regularly-scheduled service of remembrance (or memorial service), honoring residents who are recently deceased. Depending on the facility, these may be scheduled in common assembly rooms or in the chapel/synagogue at regular intervals (i.e. monthly or quarterly), or shortly after a particular resident's death. As part of a facility's ongoing religious program, such a service can be an important source of spiritual comfort and strength to other residents. Not only does it allow them to express their own grief over the loss of fellow residents, but it also reinforces the knowledge that they too will be remembered by others after they have passed from this world. Moreover, it also gives staff an opportunity to honor the memories of residents with whom they worked and grew close, and this can be particularly important when they cannot attend the actual funerals.

A facility-sponsored service of remembrance may also help the grieving process of family members, especially if the service is held within a short time after the resident's death. When positive memories of the deceased are warmly and respectfully offered by other residents and staff, families may draw additional solace from the knowledge that their loved ones were appreciated and valued within the SRC community. Moreover, any friction that remains between a resident's family and staff may be eased by such a gesture that promotes reconciliation and renewed good will – certainly a goal within the purview of the Jewish chaplain in both his/her priestly and pastoral roles. When services of remembrance are a part of a facility's ongoing religious program, they become a significant way to mark sacred time in the life of that facility

---

13   For more on ceremonies of welcoming, cf. Cary Kozberg, "Let Your Heart Take Courage: A Ceremony for Entering a Nursing Home", *A Heart of Wisdom*, edited by Susan Berrin, 1997, Jewish Lights Publishing, pp. 289-297 and "Let Your Heart Take Courage", *Aging and Spirituality,* Vol. 6, No. 4, Winter 1994.

and thereby further promote *kedushah*/sanctity by strengthening the sense of "caring community" among residents, staff and families.[14]

Food, Ethnicity And Sanctity: The Importance Of Kosher

According to Frank Podietz, retired CEO of Abramson Care Center in Philadelphia, there are two things that make a Jewish-sponsored SRC facility authentically "Jewish": the presence of a Jewish chaplain and the observance of *kashrut*, the Jewish dietary laws. But while pastoral care is often a part of the larger multi-disciplinary program in many SRCs (particularly those that are faith-based) only *Jewish* facilities – by definition – maintain kosher kitchens and provide exclusively kosher food to their residents. Since *kashrut* (the Jewish dietary laws) is an abiding and tangible symbol of Jewish religion and culture, it follows that when Jews for whom these dietary laws are important choose a senior residential care setting, that setting's being "kosher" will be a key factor. Thus, from a marketing perspective, *kashrut* may be an important form of "branding".[15]

Even for Jews who themselves may pay little attention to the religious/spiritual reasons and meaning of these laws, a place that is "kosher" often means that its population and ambience will be reliably "Jewish" and therefore culturally and ethnically familiar to them.[16] But whether from a cultural perspective or a religious one, observance of the kosher laws is still believed to be a basic necessity in making a

---

14   For more on the importance of resident memorial services, cf. Sheila Segal's chapter, "Grief and Mourning in Senior Residential Care: A Jewish Pastoral Framework".

15   To be sure, it is also argued that the absence of *kashrut* is also an important form of "branding". In order to attract Jews for whom *kashrut* is not important and to keep operating costs down, some Jewish SRCs are moving away from a "kosher-only" policy. Cf. Nathaniel Popper, "Bowing to Market, Consumer Demand, Some Jewish Nursing Homes Go Treyf", *Forward,* January 27, 2010.

16   This is certainly not to imply that SRCs not under Jewish auspices are unable to meet the religious/cultural needs of their Jewish residents. On the contrary, chapters in this book by Rabbis Sharon Mars, Beverly Magidson and Rev. Jim Jensen attest to the opposite. While they are certainly not expected to have kosher kitchens, non-Jewish SRCs that are sensitive to the particular needs of their Jewish residents can and do make arrangements for obtaining kosher food when it is requested.

Jewish SRC "a *Jewish* home", and not just a home where Jewish people live.[17] In facilities where this belief is affirmed, a key responsibility of a Jewish chaplain in a Jewish SRC is to advocate that the Jewish dietary laws continue to be observed. Such advocacy may include educating residents, staff and families about its significance, while addressing any challenges that may hamper the integrity of their observance.

The challenges can be significant. While *kashrut* is part and parcel of the Jewish *communal* ethos, individual Jews are not necessarily committed to its observance.[18] Some may regard this part of Jewish life as merely a historical memory, a carry-over from a distant past with no real significance in today's world. Others may believe (wrongly) that the dietary laws were originally promulgated for hygienic reasons. Their argument is that, with modern food preparation methods and sanitation, they are no longer necessary. Moreover, because the rules themselves involve focus and precision, they are often dismissed as too confusing and too cumbersome to bother with.

In addition, there are added material and labor expenses associated with providing kosher food. Maintaining a kosher kitchen that serves dozens (or hundreds) of people three meals a day, 365 days a year, involves significantly extra cost and effort. Besides the extra expense of kosher meat and poultry (which involves slaughtering animals in a particular way, after which the animal's blood must be thoroughly removed through a specific method)[19] there is the need to keep "meat" and "dairy" separate. Whenever meat or poultry is served, food items containing milk or milk products may be not served, and *vice versa*. This refers not only to food products, but also to dishes, utensils, cookware etc. used in preparation and serving.[20]

---

17   Again, this belief is not universally held. Cf. note 14 above and the letters written in response to Popper's article by Rabbi Sara Paasche Orlow, Linda M. Sterthous, and Rabbis Cary Kozberg and James Michaels. *Forward* February 17, 2010.

18   Cf. notes 14 and 16.

19   This millennia-old process is called *sh'chitah*, and the person who does the slaughtering is called a *shochet*. The requirement of blood removal is based on Genesis 9:4.

20   The prohibition against mixing meat and dairy is based on Exodus 23:19, 34:26 and Deuteronomy 14:21. That this commandment appears three separate times in Scripture was an indication for the Talmudic sages of its extreme importance, to which they responded with additional interpretation

Because of the need for focus and precision for proper observance, most Jewish SRCs that are "certified kosher" usually have a *mashgiach* (supervisor/overseer) on site to make sure that things are done properly. Sometimes the chaplain may also be the facility's *mashgiach*, with the additional responsibility of direct, hands-on *kashrut* supervision. However, a more preferable arrangement is when a facility either employs, or contracts with, an individual whose sole responsibility is *kashrut* supervision. This entails overseeing that all food purchases and preparation are within kosher guidelines, making sure that a proper separation between "meat" and "dairy" is maintained, as well as offering on-going education to staff about matters pertaining to *kashrut*. And because most facility staff (both those who work in dining services and those involved in direct patient care) may begin their employment with little or no knowledge of this subject, such on-going education is necessary in order to maximize their knowledge and commitment, while trying to minimize ignorance and apathy.

Given the challenges of extra expense, added effort, ignorance and apathy, and the occasional ridiculing comment, why should Jewish SRCs continue to maintain *kashrut* as part of their programs? Why should they continue to devote so much energy and so many resources into what many consider to be a perennial operational headache, particularly when resources are increasingly scarce and there are so many other issues on which to focus?

The answer is simply this: even with the necessary extra attention and resources that *kashrut* requires, the Jewish community, as a *faith community*, continues to affirm its necessity not only as a religious obligation, but also as a privilege. Aside from the ethnic/cultural significance of *kashrut*, and the "branding" advantage it may afford when marketing to the Jewish community, the regimen itself is a tangible and ever-present symbol of the *kedushah*/sanctity that Jewish SRCs are religiously mandated to nurture. Again, maintaining *kashrut* is one important way that they participate in the larger Jewish community's covenantal mandate to promote *kedushah*/sanctity in the world – which is the reason given by Scripture for these laws in the first place![21]

---

and expansion. For a concise treatment of the laws of *kashrut*, cf. Samuel H. Dresner and Seymour Siegel, *The Jewish Dietary Laws*, 1966, New York: Burning Bush Press, and Isaac Klein, *A Guide to Jewish Religious Practice*, 1979, New York: JTS, pp. 301-378.

21   According to Scripture, although the first food restriction incumbent

The "Pastoral" Role

Older people need a vision, not only recreation.
Older people need a dream, not only a memory.
It takes three things to attain a sense of significant being:
God, a soul, and a moment. And the three are always here.[22]

As noted above, a significant challenge of old age is experiencing the loss of physical health and vitality, loss of physical attractiveness, loss of loved ones, and loss of status. Individuals who become residents of SRCs will also face the challenge of responding to the (at least partial) loss of independence and personal autonomy. These losses are often accompanied by feelings that include, but are not limited to:

- *Anger* ("How could my family/God do this to me?")
- *Unproductiveness/uselessness* ("What good am I now to anyone?")
- *Abandonment* ("I've been left here to die. Where are my family/ friends? Where is God?")

Such feelings contribute to a person's feeling significantly diminished and increasingly alienated. Indeed, this increased sense of alienation is exacerbated by the standards of a culture which values activity, youth, and productivity, a culture in which living in a senior residential center is not seen as "living", but is not yet death (no wonder residents may feel they are in "God-forsaken" places!). Thus, the underlying existential question for such individuals becomes: *what does my life mean now … if anything?* Again, trying to find meaning, a "sense of sameness" and maintain a sense of personal identity and integrity of self, SRC residents (and their families) are often challenged to confront

---

upon all humanity appears in Genesis 9:4 with the prohibition against eating the blood of an animal, this restriction is given in the context of a Divine concession: part of God's covenant with all humanity after the Flood, was allowing human beings to eat animal flesh. Later, as part of God's call to the Jewish people to be holy and separate from other nations, additional food restrictions were given to them as a symbol of this holiness and separation. Cf. Exodus 19:5-6 and Leviticus 19:2, 20: 25-26. For references to which animals are/are not permitted, cf. Leviticus 11: 2-47, Deuteronomy 14:3. For references to the need to separate "meat" and "dairy", see previous note.

22   Heschel, p. 82.

the burden of empty time and the tyranny of routine – time that passes without meaning and thus without hope.[23]

Chaplains conduct formal worship and life-passage rituals in the context of their "priestly" role. However, these rituals can also be effective tools to be utilized as they serve in their "pastoral" role. Serving in a pastoral capacity, the chaplain focuses specifically on the individual – on his/her particular circumstances, on feelings of despair and abandonment, as well as on the concerns of family members.[24] If it is true that "old age is often an age of anguish and … the only answer to such anguish is a *sense of significant being*,"[25] the chaplain is often the professional not only designated to help those in anguish achieve and maintain this sense of "significant being", but also affirm that this significance is based on the belief that *all* human beings, created in God's image, have infinite worth, no matter what their circumstances or condition.

Just as the chaplain-as-priest helps maintain residents' connections to the faith community as it marks sacred time and connects to God through ritual and ceremony, so the chaplain-as-pastor represents God's presence and concern to the individual. He/she works to restore a sense of hope among those who are struggling and hurting, inviting them to partake of Divine compassion and empathy, particularly when they are feeling despair and abandoned by people and by God. The chaplain's pastoral presence brings the age-old prophetic message of God's caring: "*Fear not, for I am with you; be not frightened for I am your God; I will strengthen you and I will help you; I will uphold you with My power.*"[26]

As part of the interdisciplinary care team, the chaplain may respond to concerns that are not only spiritual, but also psycho-social in nature. As such, his/her efforts may intersect with those of the team's social worker. Writing about chaplaincy in Jewish long-term care settings, Rabbi Gary Lavit points out that even though the concerns of the chaplain and the social worker may overlap, the role of the chaplain is distinctly different from that of the social worker, just as it differs from that of a "non-chaplain" rabbi ("Rav").

Lavit suggests that, rather than starting with "the religious Text"

---

23   Friedman, pp. 362-363.

24   Cf. Leonie Nowitz and Naomi Mark's chapter, "Jewish Spiritual Help for Family Caregivers".

25   Heschel, ibid., p. 77 (italics his).

26   Isaiah 41:10.

(understood to represent God's will for the community) and a concern to bring people in compliance with the Text, the chaplain begins with the person, who is "the living human document". He/she brings learning/ wisdom and skill from diverse resources to the moment: religious teachings, psychological training, the person's own background, as well as from the chaplain's own personhood.[27]

In addition to helping residents solve practical problems related to living in SRCs, the social worker also works to help with residents' psychological or emotional issues. In so doing, he/she also shares the perspective that places the person at the center, usually working from a value-neutral, "non-judgmental" stance. The chaplain, on the other hand, represents a religious tradition that affirms ethical behavior as sacred, with clear notions of what is right and what is wrong. The social worker helps individuals deal with difficult emotions in ways that are non-threatening and non-judgmental. He/she validates the person out of an "unconditional positive regard", being careful not to express approval or disapproval of the person's feelings or behaviors. The chaplain may also validate the person out of the same positive regard, perhaps also taking care not to judge what the person says or does. But as Lavit suggests, when the chaplain is listening and responding, there is an implication that God somehow is listening and responding. Thus, when the person is telling the chaplain his/her story – with accompanying fears and struggles – there is a sense that there are not just two entities in the conversation, but also an unseen Third.

With this in mind, the chaplain brings another resource that is both expected of, and unique to his/her discipline: prayer. While formal worship and the recitation of standard liturgical and biblical passages may be helpful at specific times (when offered by the chaplain in the "priestly" role), prayer facilitated spontaneously by the chaplain brings an affirmation of "sacred caring" to the anguished moment. When

---

27   Rabbi Gary Lavit, quoting Anton Boisen, in "The Difference between Chaplain, Social Worker and Rabbi", unpublished essay, p. 1. Also, cf. Rabbi Dayle Friedman, "PaRDeS: Compassionate Spiritual Presence With Elders", *Jewish Visions For Aging*, 2008, Jewish Lights Publishing, pp. 130-144. Based on the idea of person as "living document", Rabbi Friedman offers a theory of pastoral care based on the template of textual analysis suggested by the 13th-century rabbi and mystic, Rabbi Moses deLeon, called **PaRDeS**. In this system, each letter (consonant) represents a level of textual understanding/ interpretation, progressing from the most literal / "factual" to the most profound/ spiritual, corresponding to the levels of relating to the individual.

individualized in the context of the pastoral one-on-one encounter, it can be spiritually therapeutic and healing. In such circumstances the experience of praying – of connecting to God – must "fit" the needs of the resident at that moment, and the chaplain must know how and when to make it fit properly.[28]

The importance of knowing how and when to appropriately respond to residents is nowhere more evident than in working with residents who are cognitively impaired. The chaplain must also be available for these individuals – arguably even more so than for others. Ours is a "hyper-cognitive" culture, in which individuals are valued and honored because of productivity based on their cognitive and rational abilities. In such a culture, a person's worth and dignity fade as these abilities disappear. In such a culture, it is often also assumed that when cognitive capacity diminishes, so does one's capacity to connect spiritually.

For staff members who work with these residents, however, nothing could be further from the truth. In all sorts of ways, religious and non-religious, persons with dementia, are able to demonstrate (if not cogently articulate) a spirituality that is often alive and vibrant – sometimes more vibrant when the filter of "cognition" has weakened. Representing the truth that God cares about, and is present to all creatures – regardless of how well their brains work – the chaplain offers a "ministry of presence".[29] Whereas a person's conventional/"normal" responses in a pastoral encounter depend on memory, reason, cognitive integration, some or all of these capacities are usually weaker or totally absent in persons with cognitive impairment. In these circumstances, a ministry of presence is simply that: being "fully present", and focusing on the person in that particular moment and not on the presenting "problem". When a person's verbal responses are no longer cogent, a ministry of presence listens more to the "melody" – tone of voice, body language – and less to the "lyrics"/actual words. Denying that persons with dementia have been forsaken by God, a ministry of presence communicates with eye contact and touch (when appropriate) *safety* and *total acceptance*: "I am here for you and I care about you." Indeed, because persons with dementia intuitively know when someone does or does not care about

---

28   For more on the history of spontaneous prayer in Jewish tradition and its efficacy in Jewish pastoral care, cf. Gary Lavit's chapter, "Jewish Spontaneous Prayer: The Blessings and the Challenges".

29   Henri J.M. Nouwen, *The Wounded Healer*, 1972, Garden City: Doubleday, p. 65 ff.

them, the authenticity the chaplain brings to this type of encounter is essential: it is what ultimately creates connections that are "soul to soul."[30] It is these kinds of connections that create a *kedushah*/sanctity which is uniquely "awe-ful" in the midst of a reality that is, for most people, uniquely dreadful.

The last (but decidedly not least) for whom the chaplain as pastoral caregiver must be available are the facility's staff. Again, unlike the social worker whose focus is almost always solely on residents and their families, the chaplain may be called upon to offer pastoral care and support to fellow employees who are struggling with issues at work or in their personal lives. Whether the issue is a difficult resident/family member or an unsympathetic supervisor, an abusive spouse or an empty checking account, whether the need requires a vocal advocate or simply a listening ear, the chaplain needs to be responsive. He/she must be available and willing to help resolve the issues staff members bring to the best of his/her ability – and always within the boundaries of the facility's policies.

The chaplain's not sharing the same religious faith as his colleagues should not make a difference, particularly if the chaplain is known to be approachable, empathic and above all, trustworthy in keeping confidences. In a Jewish SRC in which most staff are not only not Jewish, but may have either little prior knowledge or even negative attitudes about Jews and Judaism, the Jewish chaplain's attitudes and responsiveness (or lack thereof) may certainly affect staff members' personal attitudes and feelings.

This is one reason why the importance of "one-on-one" pastoral care again cannot be overstated. Personally speaking, experience has taught me that the Jewish chaplain relates most effectively to non-Jewish staff when he/she can relate not as clergy to layperson and not as Jew to non-Jew, but as one human being to another: laughing and rejoicing together in good times, struggling and mourning together in sad times. By being available and staying authentic, the chaplain affirms his/her

---

30   Marty Richards, "Spiritual Care for the Cognitively Impaired", presentation at ASA Conference, March 13, 1992, quoted in Rabbi Cary Kozberg, "As the Spirit Moves…", *Journal of Geriatric Care Management*, Vol. 18, No. 2, Fall 2008, p. 23.

For more on how Jewish tradition responds to the challenge of dementia, cf. also Ellen Cahn's chapter "Judaism and Dementia", and Rabbi Dayle Friedman "Seeking the Tzelem", *Jewish Visions*, pp. 38-57.

fellow workers as people. Moreover he/she also role-models how to better care for others unconditionally, so that they might do the same for those under their care. In this way, the chaplain teaches how one might serve as a better, more faithful "deputy shepherd" – and thus bring more *kedushah*/sanctity into the workplace.

The "Pedagogic" Role

Scripture relates that God's call to the community of Israel at Mount Sinai to be "a kingdom of priests and a holy people" occurred just before He spoke the Ten Commandments (Exodus 19: 5-6). From this call, the faith community of Israel has always understood that in order to fulfill its mandate to promote *kedushah*/sanctity and affirm God's presence in the world, it must constantly learn Torah and be engaged in the kinds of behavior that Torah expects.

Since those expectations are not always manifestly clear from what Scripture states, simply "reading the Word" is never sufficient; it must also be discussed, debated and interpreted in order to make it continually speak to the community. This is the responsibility of rabbis – Judaism's recognized religious authorities. For this reason, the word "Torah" does not refer only to the five books of Moses, but also to the rest of Hebrew Scripture AND to the legal and homiletic interpretations offered by the rabbinic sages over the centuries. In short, whatever recognized religious authorities learn and teach in any given time is considered to be "Torah", and *Talmud Torah* (learning Torah) as a life-long activity is a supreme act of piety.

For older adults, particularly those who reside in SRCs, engaging in *talmud Torah* has an added significance. Commenting on the revelation at Sinai, the rabbinic sages taught that when God spoke to Israel, every person present heard the Voice, each according to his/her own abilities: the wise heard it in their way, the simple in their way; men heard it in their way, women heard it in their way; the young heard it in their way, and the elderly in their way. Everyone heard the Voice uniquely, perhaps because the hearing was primarily not just a sensory experience, but a spiritual one.[31] In the role of "teacher", the Jewish chaplain helps residents continue to "hear the Voice". In various formal and informal,

---

31   *Midrash Tanhuma*, Exodus 25, quoted in *Sefer Aggadah: Legends from the Talmud and Midrash*, edited by H. N. Bialik and Y. H. Ravitzky, 1992, New York: Schocken, p.80.

but always creative, ways he/she helps them to maintain their intellectual and spiritual connections to the best of their abilities. He/she works to steer them away from the ever-present possibility of mental stagnation and spiritual alienation by offering ongoing opportunities to continue (or even begin!) to have a meaningful interface with the teachings of Judaism, so that the end of their lives will still have opportunities for increasing wisdom and nurturing spiritual growth.[32]

I am intentionally using the phrase "have a meaningful interface" instead of the word "learn", because what the chaplain does in the role of pedagogue must of course be meaningful to residents, but in ways that offer more than merely sponsoring religious intellectual activities. Certainly, formal classes and informal discussions on Scripture, rabbinic literature, the Jewish prayerbook, Jewish history, customs and practices and Jewish current events are welcomed and necessary. These, along with other learning programs such as adult Bar/Bat Mitzvah or Confirmation groups, not only continue to keep minds active, but also serve to enhance personal self esteem by providing opportunities for "doing *mitzvahs*" – actively observing the commandments.[33] However, just as in the pastoral role, the chaplain's pedagogic role is also about enriching the spirit, but in a different way. Working with the facility's Activities staff, the chaplain should provide not only activities with a strong intellectual component, but also programs with a strong *affective* component. To be sure, focusing on "affect" may be more important, particularly for residents with diminished cognitive and intellectual capacities. Such activities might include programs on Jewish humor, various kinds of Jewish music, Jewish reminiscing groups, group poetry writing (having the poems published with the residents' names attached always makes them feel good!), and activities focusing on the spiritual themes of various Jewish holidays.[34] Intergenerational programs led by

---

32   For more on the importance of Torah study in senior care centers, cf. David Glicksman's chapter "Torah Study in Senior Residential Care".

33   Rabbi Dayle Friedman suggests that programs of "doing *mitzvahs*" can be effective antidotes to the problems of boredom and routine in nursing homes. Cf. her chapter "Spiritual Challenges of Nursing Home Life" in *Aging, Spirituality and Religion*, edited by M. Kimble, S. McFadden, J. Ellor and J. Seeber, 1995, Fortress Press, pp. 362-373.

34   For creative ways to combine Jewish holiday themes with rehabilitative therapies, cf. Kate Brown's chapter "Playing Dreidel: A Unique "Spin" on Combining Jewish Holidays and Rehabilitative Therapies.

a social worker and the chaplain in which residents and their families talk about the meaning of getting older and increasing dependence, as well as programs that help residents prepare ethical wills for their families and loved ones can be especially meaningful and enriching for both residents and families.[35] Others may combine presenting Jewish spiritual themes in the context of arts therapy.[36]

As a compliment to activities of a more intellectual bent, these focus more on the heart than the head. They seek to edify the spirit rather than educate the mind. While they are more suitable and helpful to those with limited intellectual abilities, they also offer benefits of a more "holistic" nature to residents who are not cognitively challenged. Including both kinds of activities in a comprehensive religious activities program will help Jewish residents continue to "hear the Voice" by keeping them connected to their religious and cultural legacy.

It goes without saying that when the population includes residents who are not Jewish, such efforts must certainly not be limited to the Jewish ones. As *the* religious resource in a Jewish-sponsored SRC, the chaplain may be approached by non-Jewish residents and their families with various questions or feedback. He/she may be asked anything from "what does 'kosher' mean" to "why don't we get therapy on Saturdays?"; from "why are you fasting today?" to "may I participate in the Torah study group, even though I'm not Jewish?". Being accessible to *everyone*, the chaplain makes Judaism more accessible, and thus continues to further the facility's mission of promoting *kedushah*/sanctity.[37]

Such availability is also tremendously important when it comes to working with the facility's staff. As both teacher and counselor to staff, the chaplain is there to help promote a better understanding of the religious nature of the facility's ethos and work environment, as well as how Judaism relates to, or affects the particulars of their specific jobs. This is a major reason why the chaplain must participate in orienting and acclimating new staff; he/she is usually the best person to articulate the "Jewish" mission of the facility to new employees – some of whom very

---

35   Cf. Josh Stanton's and Hedy Peyser's chapter "Lessons for Living: Creating Ethical Wills in Senior Residential Care Settings".

36   Cf. Deborah Delsignore's chapter. "A Picture's Worth 1000 Souls: Partnering Creative Arts Therapy and Jewish Spiritual Care."

37   Cf. my chapter "For You Know the Heart of the Stranger: Addressing the Spiritual and Religious Needs of Non-Jewish Residents in Jewish Senior Residential Care Venues".

likely will have no prior knowledge or experience of Jews or Judaism.

This "introduction to Judaism" at orientation should be followed by periodic in-service sessions that focus on the various religious/spiritual/cultural aspects of Judaism. Geared to the entire staff or to specific departments, topics may include:

- The importance and specifics of *kashrut*.
- Jewish holiday observances (what they mean and what staff need to know *viz*. changes in daily routine, assistance with holiday observances, etc.).
- Jewish ethical approaches to end-of-life issues.
- Understanding the dynamics of Jewish families and how to better respond to them (helpful as part of a wider training in diversity).

Even as the Jewish chaplain is mindful to highlight the differences between Judaism and other religious faiths when appropriate, he/she can also highlight religious similarities. This can be done by offering informal (and completely voluntary) Bible study sessions and/or workshops promoting spirituality in the workplace – both crafted with clearly articulated ecumenical intent and open to all staff. Such programs may also serve to strengthen religious commonalities among staff (not to mention the chaplain's own visibility).[38] In addition, the chaplain will certainly want to be involved in programs that help staff better understand the unique situations of residents who are Holocaust survivors, so that they can address issues that may arise with this special population with more sensitivity.[39] And if the facility itself is a site where formal clinical training is offered to other chaplains working in senior residential care settings, the chaplain's participation and "Jewish input" will certainly be of significance.[40]

---

38   For more on promoting a deeper sense of spirituality among senior residential care staff, cf. *Vital Connections in Long Term Care*, edited by Julie Barton, Marita Grudzen and Ron Zielske, 2003, Health Care Press.

39   Cf. Paula David's chapter, "More Battles: Age-Related Challenges for Holocaust Survivors". Besides inviting outside speakers, arranging a staff trip to a Holocaust museum can be quite powerful in helping staff to better understand, intellectually and emotionally, what happened during that time, as well as the magnitude, depth and long-term effects of the suffering it caused.

40   Cf. Sara Paasche-Orlow's chapter, "Professional Development in

The "Prophetic" Role

Judaism teaches that there are two ways in which *kedushah*/sanctity increase in the world: 1) when humans perform certain duties focusing on God, and 2) when they perform certain duties focusing on their fellows. The first is usually associated with fulfilling the commandments pertaining to ritual observance, while the second is usually associated with acting ethically, morally and compassionately toward others.

It is axiomatic that the second always has the first in mind: when we behave ethically and compassionately toward our fellows, we are doing what God wants us to do. Loving God means loving His creatures; one cannot love God when one does not treat others in this way. This truth was echoed by Jesus when he reminded his listeners that the two greatest commandments are "Love the Lord your God" and "Love your neighbor as yourself", and that "on these two commandments hang all the Law and the prophets".[41]

In ancient Israel, the role of the prophets was largely to remind the people that only through ethical and moral behavior could the community realize its covenantal mandate to be a "kingdom of priests and a holy nation". This message was not especially popular, especially when conventional wisdom taught (and somehow still does) that true religious behavior has everything to do with ritual observance and little to do with interpersonal behavior. Nevertheless, the prophets of old said what needed to be said, often under pain of bodily harm or threat of death, believing that it was their God-given duty (literally), from which they could not desist. In this way, they were the conscience of their society and culture.

This is the context out of which the chaplain functions in the "prophetic" role. Just as the prophets were the ethical (and thus religious) conscience of ancient Israel, so chaplains are the conscience of the care facilities in which they serve. They personify the mission and values statements of the institution. As such, their role in giving input to both the administration and board of directors is crucial. As Nathan the prophet was both ally and goad to King David, so the chaplain's role is to both support and challenge policies and decisions. Knowing when each is needed and appropriate, the chaplain must also remind his/her superiors and colleagues that both support and challenge are

---

Geriatric Chaplaincy: Revealing the Jewish Voice".

41   Matthew 22:33-40; Mark 12: 28-31.

legitimate aspects of this particular role.

At the same time, just as the prophets of Israel had to be both "for" God and the people simultaneously when the two were at odds with one another, the chaplain may also have to be "for" two opposing parties at the same time when there are points of conflict between them: administration vs. staff, staff vs. staff, staff vs. resident(s), resident(s) vs. staff, resident(s) vs. administration … even resident vs. resident's family. Representing the ethical principles while needing to be supportive of all parties (but not necessarily all positions), the chaplain as "prophet" must also advocate that all interactions among people within the facility – written or spoken, casual or otherwise – consistently follow the religious rules of ethical speech.

In Jewish tradition, complying with the rules of ethical speech is a universal expectation of huge religious significance. It is an essential way of promoting *kedushah*/sanctity in the real world. Combining both the "pedagogic" and "prophetic" roles, the chaplain is in a unique position to teach staff about what these rules entail – rules about gossip, truth-telling (is it always appropriate, even ethical?), offering praise/giving criticism (essential in doing evaluations) – as well as help with their implementation. In this way, his/her input and influence can make a huge impact on a facility's work environment and staff morale.

Moreover, the chaplain must be able to "speak truth" to both the powerful and the not-so-powerful, while staying mindful of how feelings of fear, personal affection or pity may unduly influence or compromise his/her position. The chaplain must be able to express support when necessary, and also appropriately challenge when necessary (albeit gently, yet firmly). As one housekeeper once put it, "Rabbi, we want and expect you to 'keep it real'!"

But "keeping it real" calls for levels of both professional and personal integrity that are, by definition, "above average". Along with the knowledge and familiarity of Jewish sources, such integrity is essential for the chaplain to be the institution's main moral/ethical voice when hard clinical and/or administrative decisions need to be made: whether or not therapy should be offered on the Sabbath and holy days (with the facility possibly losing revenue); whether or not a resident's artificial feeding should be stopped, or a chronically verbally-abusive resident be evicted.[42] Just as we imagine that God is

---

42   More on the chaplain's role in ethical decision making in Rabbi James Michaels' chapter, "The Ethics Committee as a Venue for Pastoral Care".

"dynamic", constantly moving between the attribute of Strict Justice and the attribute of Undeserved Compassion, so the prophetic role of the chaplain is dynamic – he/she must often take positions between these two opposites. And when, in any given situation, the chaplain is called to work in a "prophetic" capacity, he/she must do so, being ever mindful of the other three roles.

A Fifth "P": Presence

Can persons in the end live without a sense of the sacred? Do we inevitably discover sacredness in (or ascribe sacredness to) something central to our lives as persons and societies?[43]

For people of faith, the answer to the first question is "no", while the answer to the second would seem to be "we are able to discover sacredness, but it is not inevitable that we do". It is true that senior residential care settings are often described as "dreadful," "frightening," and "loathsome." Experiencing *kedushah* and a sense of the sacred in what are often considered to be "God forsaken places" is indeed very difficult for many people. But while it may be difficult, it is not impossible.

In their younger years, it is unlikely that most individuals even *think* about the notion of "sanctity", much less seek it out. But as they age, adults often begin to pay more attention to spiritual matters and improving their "inner lives", and come to better appreciate experiences which we would call "sacred". Moreover, when aging is accompanied by frailty and physical and/or cognitive loss, the quest for meaning and a "sense of something" that will transcend the residents' own lives may become more urgent.

That the general mandate to "be holy"[44] includes a specific commandment to pay deference and show honor to the elderly,[45] clearly shows Scripture's sensitivity to this phenomenon. Working in the various roles described above, the Jewish chaplain strives to epitomize this mandate.

Alluded to and demonstrated throughout this chapter, it is often

---

43   Alan Mittelman, "Asking the Wrong Question", *First Things*, No. 189, January, 2009, p. 17.

44   Leviticus 19:2.

45   Leviticus 19:32.

the chaplain's presence *alone* – and not any role or task he/she performs
– that often inspires residents to continue hold on to hope and purpose
by bearing witness to the religious truth that God has *not* forsaken these
places.

Over the years, colleagues have shared many stories from their
work affirming the symbolic power of the chaplain's pastoral presence.
One particularly poignant example happened to my co-editor Jim
Michaels. He tells of a 97-year-old man who, although legally blind,
lived for several years in an independent living facility. After a series
of emotional traumas, this gentleman was unable to walk, feed, or care
for himself and moved into the long-term care facility where Rabbi
Michaels is the chaplain. For more than a year, he remained on his unit,
rarely going to any of the many activities that were offered. Whenever
Rabbi Michaels came to visit other residents, he always said hello to
this resident, but their interactions were rarely more than the social
niceties.

During a visit by the rabbi to his unit on December 31, 2009, the
man called him over and said he wanted to start attending religious
services. "It's my new year's resolution," he said. He meant what he said
and began attending almost daily. Working with a physical therapist, he
gained enough strength and mobility to ambulate his way to and from
the synagogue, despite his near total vision impairment.

Two years later, the man's daughter encountered Rabbi Michaels
in the lobby and invited him to a 100th birthday party for her father
that was soon to take place. Then she thanked him for "all you've
done," explaining that it was due to *his* intervention that her father
had made so much progress. Of course, Rabbi Michaels had really done
nothing specific or tangible for the man; he had only been a symbolic
presence for him. While any number of factors might have contributed
to the improvement of his physical and emotional demeanor, it was
the chaplain's symbolic but powerful pastoral presence which played
such a significant role in his progress and decision to continue not to
give up.[46]

Jewish tradition teaches that as a sign of God's never-failing love
and concern for the people of Israel, the *Shekhinah* (God's Presence)
accompanied them into exile throughout their history and waits with

---

46   For more on the subject of how a rabbi's symbolic role serves as the
source of his/her authority and power, cf. *The Rabbi As Symbolic Exemplar: By
the Power Vested in Me*, 2002, Haworth Press.

them for the final Redemption.[47] Recalling this teaching, we may understand it as a metaphor for the symbolic, yet powerful presence of the chaplain as he/she accompanies residents, families and staff in their own "exiles" and struggles with loss, disconnection, frustration. The presence of Jewish chaplains – serving in all their roles as ever-faithful "deputy shepherds" – attests not to God's absence in senior care facilities, but rather to His ever-abiding proximity.

Keeping this tenet in the forefront of their facilities' culture and ethos, they hold up to everyone who walks through the doors this truth: "just *to be* is a blessing; just *to live* is holy."[48]

---

47   Babylonian Talmud, Megillah. 29a; Zohar 1:120b.
48   Heschel, ibid., p. 84.

Chapter 2
Dependence And Empowerment: Jewish Approaches And Responses

Rabbi Daniel Coleman

Long before Americans began to celebrate Independence Day and uphold symbols of freedom such as the Statue of Liberty and the Liberty Bell, Judaism affirmed the importance of liberty and independence through its holidays and rituals. For example, Sukkot and Passover celebrate the exodus from enslavement in Egypt and journey to the Land of Israel; the festivities of Purim and the lights of Hanukah celebrate freedom of religious practice. Freedom is a reminder of the capacity to be Godlike: Just as God is free so must we strive to achieve and retain our freedom. Furthermore, Judaism encourages its adherents to utilize freedom in order to become partners with God in creation. As we grow older, our ability to actualize these ideals of freedom and independence is often impacted by circumstances beyond our control, such as loss of mobility, loss of physical and/or cognitive ability, and/or the loss of strength and energy to contribute to, care for family, society, and even self. How do we as professionals assist elderly Jews in coming to terms with "being dependent" when their religion and society uphold *independence* as a primary virtue? How do we work with the elderly to reconcile the time in their lives when they lose the ability to be as creative and as productive as they once were?

Certainly there are no easy answers to this question. To be cognizant of the fact that you will never be the same – that you will never be "you" again – is more than a minor shock to the system. Such a "loss of self" is significant loss, very much like a death. Perhaps as one of one of my rabbinic colleagues suggests, such people should say *Kaddish*, the traditional mourner's prayer, for the death of who they were, while symbolically taking on new names for the new persons they have now become.

It is true that responses to such significant loss of ability and sense of self may very well include questioning G-d and/or lamenting one's circumstances – which Judaism accepts and affirms as authentic responses. One only has to look to Scripture to find that many biblical characters questioned the Holy One at some point in their lives, and that the measure of a prophet's greatness (think Abraham, Moses, Jonah) was defined by a passionate, sometimes angry, dialogue with God regarding a perceived injustice.[1] As a chaplain, I have found that the best thing I can do when someone is questioning or lamenting is simply listen, accept and validate what the person is saying. As my teacher Yehoshua Engelman eloquently put it: "The Almighty doesn't need a defense attorney. If you are on God's side, you aren't on the side of the people."

The Power Of Peer Support

Residents in senior care settings and their family members often appreciate encouragement and validation of their expressions of inadequacy, loss, uselessness, frustration and anger. Certainly, this isn't limited to Jews; persons of all faiths may welcome the permission to take their cue from Biblical personalities (and even God) when expressing real feelings of anger, betrayal, regret, mistrust and abandonment. Often this is enough to lessen the intensity and anguish of an inner emotional struggle over the individual's religious or societal "right" to entertain feelings that society labels as "negative" and unacceptable.

In some places where seniors live, this validation of free expression has engendered a focus on *peer-support*. Because of their own experiences, frail individuals may be the only ones who can really listen to, and empathize with another person in similar circumstances and not talk them out of their despondent state. Residents report that simply listening to and empathizing with other residents who are also experiencing loss of self-worth and independence restores a sense of empowerment, usefulness and a feeling of contributing to the lives of others. No longer are their own hardships viewed only as a burden on

---

1   In addition to numerous biblical accounts of individuals lamenting, the Hebrew title of the biblical book *Lamentations* is *Eichah*, meaning "why?" or "how?" – reflecting the author's giving voice to communal laments over the destruction of the Holy Temple in Jerusalem and over tragedy in general.

themselves and others, since these very hardships will them to relate to the suffering of a peer. Peer-support creates a safe and nurturing environment in which a person can feel broken and detached, yet still connect with, and have an impact upon others who may have similar life experiences. And since this model is adaptable to other settings, it can and should be encouraged by professional staff or established in places where there is no professional on hand.

Another effective form of peer-support (and) enlists the help of fellow residents to perform acts of kindness (*g'milut chasadim*) which are hallmarks of a just and caring community.[2] In a senior residential care setting, these might include welcoming new residents (*hachnasat orchim*), visiting the sick (*bikkur cholim*) and comforting the bereaved (*nichum avelim*). Indeed, while those who visit bereaved peers may also confront their own frailty and mortality and perhaps begin a process of self-grieving, engaging in various acts of kindness enables residents to feel a greater sense of empowerment and self-worth. At a time when many older individuals report a hesitancy to develop friendships for fear that they will shortly lose one more significant person in their lives, these gestures of "reaching out" can create connections with others. Furthermore, staff and residents also benefit from the increased sense of "community" and mutual responsibility for each other, which can ease their dependence on volunteers and outside visitors.

Finding Solace In Jewish Prayers

While working at a nursing home in the Bronx, I facilitated an *Oneg Shabbat* (a reception honoring the Sabbath) on several units each Friday. During one of these programs, I noticed a new gentleman who had tears in his eyes. After the program, I asked him to tell me about himself. He said that he had served as *chazan* (cantor) of a synagogue for several decades, and that listening to me during the program had evoked feelings of grief and uselessness in him. After further a discussion with his social worker and myself he agreed to serve as my cantorial assistant at these programs. Happily, this resulted not only in his feeling more serene and uplifted, but also in creating a real joy among the other residents at seeing "one of their own" play a central role in leading a group activity.

---

2   Cf. *Pirke Avot* (Ethics of the Fathers) 1:2 and the end of Shabbat 127a in the Talmud.

In my experience, another empowering "intervention" that is appreciated by residents is the offering of spontaneous "custom-made" prayers during pastoral visits or at the end of group sessions. Because of Judaism's emphasis on a formal liturgy, such devotional spontaneity is sometimes unfamiliar to some Jewish residents. I remember one resident in our facility who expressed her anguish that the onset of macular degeneration had deprived her of the ability to read from her prayer book, and her "ailing" memory was "robbing" her of the ability to recite even the most familiar prayers by heart. She was overjoyed to learn that our ancestors prayed to God in contemplative and spontaneous ways centuries before the creation of our formal liturgy, and that our conversations with God are not dependent on being in synagogue or reciting specific words.

It is important however to acknowledge and address the feeling of loss a person may feel when he/ is no longer able to attend synagogue or express the hallowed words of his/her religious tradition, and thus feels cut off from the community. One way of responding is the creation of "prayer partners", an idea shared with me by one of my peers in my Clinical Pastoral Education (CPE) experience, Reverend Colin Baker.

Residents who participate in this program are invited to select a partner or "buddy" to whom they can speak on a regular basis. As residents offer and seek out ways to pray, they develop and strengthen empathic bonds with those around them. They may become less dependent on a religious professional or a prayer book to guide them. In addition, they may benefit greatly from the knowledge and power of bestowing a spiritual gift on another person. Some residents even report renewed faith in their ability to affect their own spiritual destiny. In assuming responsibility for the well-being of others, they feel that they are partnering with God, while retaining a degree of connection to fellow co-religionists through prayer, and thus a renewed connection to their faith community.[3]

Lessons From The Torah

Many of the lessons learned in the Torah come from recounting the journeys, struggles and challenges which the Israelites experienced on their way to the Promised Land – experiences that continue to teach

---

3   For more on the concept of spontaneous prayer in Judaism, cf. Gary Lavit's chapter "Promoting Spontaneous Prayer".

and impact us to this day. Today we would call this "journaling", another therapeutic tool that can decrease a sense of helplessness and foster more independence. By chronicling past experiences and the lessons learned from them, individuals can express in writing their feelings, fears and concerns, particularly as they approach "the valley of the shadow" (Psalm 23). Certainly one of journaling's benefits is that it may be done individually or in groups, with the professional facilitating the process as much as necessary in his/her own setting.

It should also be noted that other modes of expression such as public readings, drama and dance also lend themselves to residents' reviewing and sharing their life stories. These modalities also offer wonderful opportunities for effective self-expression, a deeper sense of accomplishment, and even a gleaning of new wisdom. When residents direct or star in the (re)creation of an earlier unpleasant life-episode, a sense of control and reconciliation with the past can be restored. Thus, as both joyous and painful moments are explored with peers and professionals, they can hopefully be assimilated and integrated into a "present" that is satisfying and meaningful.

Ethical Wills

A reflective and creative journaling process may also inspire residents to create an ethical will.[4] Ethical wills give residents an opportunity to express highlights of their life-narratives. Rather than dwell on sorrow and laments, residents can use ethical wills to bequeath spiritual and moral lessons, thus memorializing qualities by which they want to be remembered. Such documents can be kept private, shared with fellow residents or family members, or used as a starting point for conversations with a chaplain or other professionals. Expressing personal thoughts and prayers in writing gives an alternative outlet and voice to residents, particularly to those who are speech-impaired.

---

4   For more on the benefits of seniors writing ethical wills cf. Josh Stanton's and Hedy Peyser's chapter, "Lessons of a Lifetime: Creating Ethical Wills In Senior Residential Care Settings". For general information on ethical wills, go to http://www.ethicalwill.com. Also cf. Jack Riemer and Nathaniel Stampfer, *So That Your Values Live On: Ethical Wills and How to Prepare Them* (Jewish Lights Publishing).

Times And Seasons

The regularity of the Jewish calendar presents many opportunities for enrichment of residents' lives. Even those with severe dementia often respond to the ebb and flow of the seasons and festivals, as well as the weekly observance of Shabbat. Many anticipate and look forward to the traditional observances and customs that are associated with these sacred days. Happily, the messages and themes of these days may also resonate with residents in their quest to feeling more empowered.

Shabbat: Residents may find the various messages of Shabbat (the Sabbath) to be personally and deeply meaningful. For example, Jewish tradition teaches that Shabbat was the climax of God's creation and the cessation from His creating anything new. Just as we emulate God by creating and working during the week, we are also commanded every Shabbat to emulate God by *refraining* from creative activity (*melacha*). This opportunity to take "time out" enables us to appreciate our creative accomplishments and to focus on spiritual nourishment and replenishment. Jewish tradition teaches that Shabbat and the Holy Days bestow an "additional soul", an added dimension of spirituality. It may be that older persons who have ceased to be engaged in the creative activities of their youth are better able to access this additional soul, to which the rest of us have access only on these sacred days.

Drawing upon this teaching about Shabbat can help the frail elderly transform a time of inaction, helplessness and vulnerability into a time of simply "being" and appreciating, a time of truly resting and connecting with their Ultimate Source of Being. Understanding aging as an "extended sabbatical" can help older persons to use this period in their lives as a time for reflection and integration, and hopefully a deeper appreciation of their Creator and the world around them.[5]

To be sure, even with their themes of joy and celebration, the approach of Jewish holidays may also exacerbate feelings of dejection and despair. This may be because of the importance accorded to the various home-based rituals associated with these holidays, as well as the considerable status often accorded to those who lead or facilitate them. Residents who once relished leading family and friends in the Passover Seder or Hanukah candle-lighting may indeed experience a loss of purpose and status when they realize that they are no longer

---

5   Note how closely this notion parallels Erik Erikson's idea that the primary task of those of advanced age is "life review".

able to fulfill these roles. Women may mourn the loss of their role as homemaker, particularly if they were responsible for preparing the festive meals which are central to the celebration of so many Jewish holidays (although, truth be told, many are often glad to be relieved of the responsibility). Thus, during these holidays – when the "sweet" and the "bitter" mingle – staff should be aware of the opportunities that are presented to address and validate the feelings with which residents and their families may struggle. What follows are several examples of how popular holiday themes can be used to facilitate reflection, integration and healing:

Passover: "*Dayenu*" (It would have been enough) is a well-known song that is sung at the Passover Seder table. How often do frail individuals express "Enough already! How much longer do I have to go on like this?" – a cry of despair often accompanied by anger towards anyone who lacks empathy for their predicament? Certainly we professionals should be sensitive and empathetic; we should be able to understand the resident's predicament from his/her perspective, and imagine how we might feel if we had lived purposeful and successful lives, only now to be denied continued health independence and more opportunities to leave our mark on this world.

Whenever I conduct a pre-Passover model Seder, I invite each resident to lead a section or song during the Seder. This can be an empowering experience, as residents are shown how they can still play a vital role in the traditions and rituals of their people. An individual simply sharing what song means to him/her can be quite empowering for that person. I often ask residents to share what the song *Dayenu* means to them individually. Several are surprised to hear that others feel similar feelings of anger and frustration. Yet, hearing common responses makes feel less alone and perhaps somewhat less guilty for harboring the sentiments that surface. In a more intimate setting, such a discussion be an ideal point to conduct a life-review that supports and validates different stages and milestones of residents' lives.

Hanukah: The Festival of Lights offers opportunities to explore significant relationships. Each night one candle (called the *shamash*) is used to light all the other flames on the eight-branched *menorah* (also called a *hanukiyah*). Residents can be invited to share how they themselves provided light to others – how they touched and affected the lives of those around them. Hopefully with such discussions, they will know that their role in spreading light, guidance, wisdom and passion to others will remain important and meaningful long after their own light fades. In addition, this holiday remembers the clash between the cultures of Judaism and Hellenism, the latter being the philosophy of ancient Greece which worshipped the body and human achievements. In contrast, Judaism has always affirmed that, regardless of achievements or productivity, every human being is inherently valuable and infinitely sacred, simply by virtue of being "created in God's image".

Rosh Hashanah: The Jewish New Year offers the chance for a new beginning – a message reiterated by the sound of the *shofar* (ram's horn) that is sounded on this holiday. But how is the loud, strong call of the *shofar* received by those who are frail? Might they be bitter or anxious about their inability to respond to its call of hope and anticipation of a more productive year ahead? Does their frailty make them all too aware of the breath that is needed to produce each *shofar* sound – an awareness that may be heightened by the use of supplementary oxygen?

It may be helpful to remind residents and their families that the rituals and prayers of Rosh Hashanah commemorate God's breathing a soul into Adam, and thus the birth of humanity as we know it. At least once a year, we pause to consider the divine breath that God continues to breath into each one of us. Such a consideration might lead to a very practical discussion about "when breathing stops" and the topic of advanced directives. It might also be wonderful pastoral and theological opportunity to discuss birth into the world and what Judaism teaches about afterlife, with sensitivity to whatever fears concerns may be expressed about end-of-life issues.

Gratitude Within The Struggle

Many Jews begin their daily prayers with the expression "*Modeh ani...*" thanking God for restoring the soul anew after overnight divine safekeeping. This theme continues in another prayer recited toward the beginning of the traditional morning service with these words: "As long as my soul is within me, I will express gratitude to You." During times when life may be viewed as a burden and consist of a string of indignities, it can be hard to be thankful for the daily gift of life. Nevertheless, Judaism encourages the cultivation of gratitude and indebtedness at every opportunity. Many Jewish prayers and blessings – like the heavenly manna that fell daily in the desert – are designed to foster an acknowledgment and an appreciation of constant dependence on God for continued sustenance and basic survival. In fact, the meaning of the name *Yehudi* (Jew) derives from the Hebrew word *modeh* – to thank and admit dependence on God.

It is noteworthy that the aforementioned expressing gratitude for the soul begins by declaring "the soul You gave me is pure: although I may not be able to do what I used to do, the part of the divine that is within me nevertheless remains pure and holy." It can be a highly empowering experience to recognize that struggling with increased dependence and becoming less active has no real substantive affect on a person's inherent value or spiritual status.

Sometimes, individuals are reluctant to inform loved ones about the debilitating nature of their ailments lest they "worry too much" or further distance themselves due to the increasing burden of care. A pastoral response might acknowledge their fears and invite residents to engage in a life-review that focuses on their experiences and challenges of taking care of others. Residents will often recall times when it was hard to provide care for someone else because the recipient was ungracious or unwilling to accept help and support. As a result, they may have felt rejected, slighted or despondent. Now that roles are reversed, the professional can help the resident find the courage to receive graciously from others.

This may be especially important when children become the parents' caregivers (providing financial, physical or emotional care and support). Perhaps it is precisely because it is so hard to accept assistance from those we raised and nurtured, that the *Torah* gives pride of place to the *mitzvah*/commandment of honoring our parents by incorporating it into the Ten Commandments. For some elderly, the knowledge (or gentle reminder) that they are continuing to help their children fulfill this important responsibility will mitigate the loss of dependence and self-worth.

Moreover, older frail individuals should be encouraged to develop a greater sense of their own worth by continuing to give to others through concrete displays of gratitude and appreciation. Examples that I often suggest include words and letters of thanks to medical staff. By contributing whatever resources are at their disposal – time, money, or simply words of praise, they can affirm the essential Jewish value of showing appreciation and gratitude. They may even begin to feel less dependent as those who give them care now become recipients of what they have to give.

We read in the book of Genesis (32:29) that God renamed Jacob "Israel" because "you wrestled with God and with man, and have prevailed". Out of that struggle, Jacob's and his descendants' identity was forever transformed. Judaism invites humanity to embrace struggle as a way of coming closer to God. This chapter has explored a number of resources that can be introduced when working with Jewish residents struggling with a loss of independence and self-worth. May God grant us the wisdom and insight to enable – and ennoble – our residents to recognize that no one can always be a doer. Sometimes we contribute simply by just "being".

Chapter 3
Jewish Spiritual Help For Family Caregivers

Leonie Nowitz, MSW and Naomi Mark, CSW

Unlike religions which emphasize "faith" over "works," Judaism underscores actions and behaviors that are rooted in religious beliefs and ideals. Jewish wisdom tradition – scriptural and later rabbinic teachings – places an exceptionally high value on actions that focus on caring for those who are vulnerable – the widow, the orphan, the sick, and the mourner. In addition to these, respecting and honoring parents and venerating the elderly are religious and moral hallmarks of all traditional Jewish communities, whose mandate is to testify to the dignity of humanity created in the divine image.

Indeed, the institution of the family is a mainstay of Jewish tradition. In a multi-generational model, every family member had a role to play. To the best of their ability, grandparents would contribute financially and help with childcare, whereas the adult children were expected to assume responsibility when their parents became old or sick. At the same time, strong traditional family ties may also affect expectations among family members, particularly when issues of geographical and/or emotional closeness or distance come into play. While older parents may expect adult children to provide needed care for them, such expectations might be difficult or sometimes impossible for the children to fulfill, due to other responsibilities of work or family, or because of geographical distance.

As noted by Rosen and Weltman,[1] the realities of modern life may

---

1   Rosen, Elliott J., and Weltman, Susan F., "Jewish Families: An Overview", in *Ethnicity and Family Therapy*, Monica McGoldrick, Joseph Giordano and Nydia Garcia–Preto, eds. 3rd Edition, 2005: The Guilford Press, p. 675.

conflict with traditional family obligations, thus causing friction between generations and exacerbating the challenges of caregiving faced by both the older parent and the adult child. In Jewish tradition, the importance of family loyalty, duty, obligation and commitment are emphasized over the value of self-fulfillment and individual choice. Yet today, with increases in life-expectancy, with a growing number of adults caring for older parents and other older family members, there are increased responsibilities – physical, emotional, and often financial commitments – placed on adult children, who themselves may belong to the cohort of people aged 50 to 70, and lead very full, albeit stressful lives.

Families struggle with the dilemma of fulfilling their commitment to care for an aging relative, while trying to fulfill other obligations to children, partners, and work. Indeed, divergent and conflicting loyalties can create a tension between a person's responsibility to parents and responsibility to one's spouse and children. This later phase of the family life cycle when parents need help often presents the challenge of constantly balancing everyone's needs. Facing such a challenge requires rethinking how to care for aging parents, who themselves may have provided for their own parents. The difficulty is increased when family members are separated by large distances.

Is it possible to preserve family unity in such circumstances? And when the question of placement in a senior residential care facility is raised, can an adult son or daughter reconcile moving a parent into such a facility with his/her own sense of caregiving obligation? Resources from Jewish tradition and culture can help family caregivers answer these questions in the affirmative.

Judaism And Filial Responsibility

Honoring one's parents is an obligation taken seriously in the Jewish tradition. The Ten Commandments contains the mandate, *Honor your father and your mother so that you may live long on the land which the Lord your God is giving you.*[2] Rabbinic commentaries interpret these words as primarily addressing the physical, material and concrete needs of one's parents and to ensure their overall well being. Significantly, the commandment is to *honor* them, but not necessarily love them: Children are obligated to behave in a respectful manner towards parents and provide for their care when necessary, regardless of personal feelings.

---

2   Exodus 20:12.

Dr. Albert Micah Lewis differentiates between ensuring that a parent receives necessary care and having to *personally* provide that care.[3] He affirms that an adult child is obligated to make sure that the parent is cared for, but is under no obligation to be the sole provider of that care. Nevertheless, it is understandable that many Jewish adult children may feel guilty when not personally providing care, given both the strong religious and societal emphases on the importance of caregiving in the Jewish tradition.

In addition, the question of how to prioritize other, possibly conflicting, needs of various family members may also be present. Jewish tradition recognizes that while individuals are commanded to care for others, they are also commanded to care for themselves and preserve their own well-being.[4] Indeed, the need to balance these two obligations was famously affirmed by the sage Hillel: "If I am not for myself, who will be for me? If I am only for myself, what am I?"[5]

Clearly, caregivers must remain aware of their own mental and physical health, knowing their own limits and despite internal high expectations. The adult child must decide when physical and/or emotional limits have been reached, and thus when to arrange for others to provide care in his/her stead.

While the decision to move a parent into a care facility may indeed be agonizing, the Jewish legal tradition recognizes the limits of an adult child's endurance, as well as limits to the availability of emotional or physical resources:

> If one's father or mother should become mentally disordered, he should try to treat them as their mental state demands, until they are pitied by God (and they die). But if he finds he cannot endure the situation because of their extreme madness, let him leave and go away, deputing others to care for them properly.[6]

The issue of financial responsibility is also discussed by rabbinical

---

3   Lewis, Dr. Albert Micah "Caring for Our Parents, Caring for Ourselves: A Jewish Perspective", in *That You May Live Long: Caring for Our Aging Parents, Caring for Ourselves*, Richard F. Address and Hara E. Person, eds. 2003: UAHC Press, p. 12.

4   Cf. Deuteronomy. 4:9.

5   *Pirke Avot* 1:14.

6   Maimonides, *Mishneh Torah, Hilkhot Mamrim* 6:10.

authorities. While some authorities hold that a child is obligated to bear the cost of a parent's needs, others argue that the child is obliged to make sure the needs are met, but may use the parent's own resources.[7] To be sure, an adult child's obligation to demonstrate honor and respect for a parent continues even after a parent is no longer residing in the family home; every act of advocacy when the parent becomes a long-term care resident is an expression of the commandment.

To summarize, Jewish tradition encourages, or even expects, adult children to "stretch hard" in order to do what is necessary to properly care for older parents. At the same time, this expectation is accompanied by certain amount of "grace" in that adult children must be able to forgive themselves, should they fall short.[8]

When Strength Begins To Fail...

Adult children of all ages find it difficult to experience their parents as vulnerable and in need of support and help when their health begins to decline. What is often experienced as a "filial crisis" is in reality a new life transition for the family: a parent's decreasing independence, accompanied by an increasing dependence on their adult children. Margaret Blenkner[9] has defined "filial maturity" as a goal that midlife adult children need to achieve when beginning to provide care to their older parents.

However, adult children are not always willing to assume the burden of caregiving and may experience a range of emotions including fear, denial and anger. One reason for this stems from our present culture's reinforcement of the denial of death. At the moment when adult children begin to notice changes in their parents' health, they may begin to confront the scary but inevitable fact that their parents will die, that they will be orphans, and that they too are mortal. While the death of a parent is a fact of life, it may nevertheless be difficult to accept and thus more easily avoided, or even denied.

---

7   Cf. Rabbi Michael Chernick, "Who Pays? The Talmudic Approach to Filial Responsibility", Address and Person, *op. cit.* pp. 95-96.

8   Rabbi Dayle Friedman, "Beyond Guilt, What We Owe Our Aging Parents – A Perspective from Tradition," Address and Person, *op. cit.* 89.

9   Blenkner M. "Social Work And Family Relationships In Later Life With Some Thoughts On Filial Maturity," *Social Structure and the Family: Generational Relations*, E Shanas and G Streib eds., 1965: Prentice Hall, pp. 46-59.

In addition, older parents may not want to admit to their own increasing limitations, resulting in both adult children and their parents colluding in denying the parents' diminishing health. This collusion comes to an abrupt end when a crisis arises. When older parents have to accept more care from their adult children, and adult children must give more care to their parents, both may struggle with this "role reversal". In such situations, flexibility, an acknowledgement of interdependence by caregivers and care-receivers – its dynamic nature, as well as an openness to change – are essential for resolution:

Mrs. M, a very proud and dignified woman in her 80s, had been living independently in her apartment and leading a fairly active life, going to classes and seeing friends, until she began to feel weaker as a result of her multiple medical challenges. Of Mrs. M's four children, only Betty lived close by. (The others lived in different cities). Although Betty worked full-time as a nurse and had children of her own, Betty also assumed responsibility for her mother's weekly grocery shopping and accompanied her mother to and from medical appointments.

Mrs. M reluctantly accepted Betty's assistance but with visible discomfort, perhaps because she viewed having to accept help in this way from her children as a diminishment of her own dignity. Betty, however, felt hurt and increasingly angry about having to shoulder the entire responsibility for her mom's care while not receiving any of the acknowledgment and "kudos" for having done so. This was especially accentuated when Mrs. M would brag to neighbors and/or her health care providers (or whomever would listen) about the wonderful accomplishments of her other children. The tension between Mrs. M and Betty escalated over the next few months. Mrs. M would complain that Betty was impatient and irritable, while Betty complained about the irony of being the designated caregiver for the parent with whom she had a strained relationship.

With the active assistance of an involved clergyman and long-time family friend who witnessed the tension during his visits, Mrs. M was helped to become a bit more complimentary and affirming towards Betty. This helped militate against Betty's understandable feelings of emotional neglect which had simmered inside her since childhood.

When Mrs. M was no longer able to live alone in the apartment, this intervention eased the adjustment for both Betty and her mom in their mutual decision to have Mrs. M move in with Betty and her family.

An important key to flexibility and openness is graciousness. While diminished independence and increasing dependence on one's children may present significant challenges to older parents, accepting assistance is easier on everyone when it is done as graciously as possible. Indeed, accepting assistance from adult children with grace and a sense of gratitude benefits the child and the parent, since it affirms their mutual interdependence.

The changes brought on by increasing dependence are multi-faceted: A child's ambivalence and anger may be rooted in wishing that parents continue to be strong, and thus always available and present, almost immortal. If the relationship has been historically strained, the adult child may be conflicted in providing care when needed. In such circumstances, professional guidance may be helpful in assisting the adult child to address and work through the issues at hand.

Even when their health is declining, many older adults prefer to live at home. (The current term for this is "aging in place.") However, placement in a residential care facility may be necessary due diminishing financial or familial resources, or deteriorating health. Certainly, if and when such a decision is made, it should be made cooperatively by adult children and the parent.

To be sure, such cooperation may not be realistic or forthcoming, and professional assistance may be necessary. Such assistance should include helping family members review together the specific circumstances at hand, how these circumstances have heretofore been handled by the family, as well as a frank discussion of the emotional cost to the family. In his/her supportive role, the professional helping such a family certainly should acknowledge their efforts while encouraging them to consider the advantages of residential care placement, as a way of better providing for the parent's increasing care needs, while also relieving the burden and stress experienced by family members.

When the transition from home to residential care does occur, family members may still feel shame and guilt, even with professional help and better communication. The older person may still feel angry and abandoned. Indeed, the transition evokes feelings of deep loss by all involved, and needs to be understood by all involved (including facility staff).

While adult children who move a parent into a residential care facility do indeed fulfill the moral and religious obligation to care for an aging parent, the manner in which this is done requires great sensitivity to both the parent's feelings and to their own. However, while sensitivity often requires time, circumstances may not permit, particularly if the move is the immediate consequence of an unplanned health crisis. Certainly, whatever anxiety or feelings of shame, guilt and displacement may accompany such a crisis these may be mitigated to some degree by intentionally discussing the possibilities of nursing home care before the need arises.

Adjusting To The Residential Care Environment: How Staff Can Help

Families accustomed to turning to older relatives for help and assistance in times of need may require additional support when those individuals are no longer in a position to assist, and securing the care of paid professionals is required. In their capacity as professional care staff, nurses, aides, social workers and pastoral care staff are expected to be sensitive to, and available to address issues and concerns of residents and family members that may arise:

Prior to Mrs. J's fall which resulted in a broken hip, she and her 42-year-old son Ben had been living together in the family home. Ben, who had been unemployed for some time, was devoted to his mother's care and catered to her every need to the extent possible. In fact, because his own life had become so focused on the care of his mom, his professional and social worlds had contracted significantly.

After Mrs. J's surgery, the interdisciplinary team and Mrs. J agreed that it would best for Mrs. J to be transferred to a rehab facility in a nursing home where she would receive the necessary care for at least several months, and perhaps long-term. Mrs. J's family – her sister and her other son – supported this plan, but Ben seemed resistant. He had developed negative impressions of the nursing home over the years, and was clearly mistrustful and suspicious of many of the aides and unit staff.

During the initial adjustment period, it became clear to the unit team that Ben's adjustment was as difficult as Mrs. J's, if not greater. After meeting with him, the social worker perceived that Ben was also suffering over the loss of his role as caregiver. Since his daily routine had revolved around caring for his mom, there was an emptiness in Ben now that he seemed to be channeling into hostility towards the staff.

The social worker arranged to have Ben included in the first few team meetings in an effort to engage him as a partner in Mrs. J's care. She made sure to seek his advice and to include him in as much decision-making as possible. She also began meeting with Ben regularly so as to provide him with the additional support during this life change.

The social worker's efforts yielded positive results. Ben responded to being treated as an important person in his mother's care and seemed to slowly begin to let go of some of the upset.

In addition to supporting family members to continue their role as caregivers by visiting and spending quality time with their loved one, encouraging both resident and family members to participate in interdisciplinary team meetings affirms the importance of their participation. It also helps staff to better discern the older person's care needs, so continuity of care can be provided. Indeed, such an approach acknowledges the fact that residential care staff and family are partners in providing care to the new resident. When family members are encouraged to visit and remain socially and emotionally available to their relatives, the transition of care responsibilities from adult children to facility staff is easier.

"I Am With You In Your Distress": Using Jewish Religious Resources

Coping with the initial transition is often quite challenging for new residents and their families. At such a time of uncertainty and anxiety, drawing upon psycho-spiritual resources, especially those provided by religious rituals, can be stabilizing and reassuring to all. Rituals, both traditional and innovative, can help provide continuity between the past and the present. They reaffirm values and a sense of purpose and also help sustain relationships within a family.

Jewish tradition marks the milestones of life, from birth to death, through various rituals and ceremonies. Because of their psycho-spiritual power, traditional rituals continue to resonate and new ones have been developed specifically to mark new transitions in later life: menopause, retirement, even the (new) phenomenon of being "empty nesters". In this spirit, some facilities offer a "welcoming ceremony" when a new resident moves in. Such a move is often a transition that truly is a "family" event. And as the family contemplates questions of what to take/what to leave behind, how life will change/be the same in the new home, family members themselves can be encouraged to participate in such a ceremony. In this way, not only can the resident be made to feel more welcomed into his/her new home, but the family also has the opportunity to feel comforted and supported in a formal but spiritually sensitive way.[10]

In planning such a ceremony for a Jewish resident, music, poetry and selections from Scripture and Jewish prayers might be included, as should well-known ritual objects such as a *kiddush* cup (used to drink wine on the Sabbath and holidays), or a *tallit* (prayer shawl). One ritual object that is especially identified with the dedication of a new dwelling is the *mezuzah*, a small, thin case with biblical verses handwritten on parchment inside; it is affixed to the right doorpost of most rooms in any Jewish home.[11]

Worshipping together can also strengthen familial and religious ties. Attending Jewish worship services is a reliable way to stay connected to the Jewish people, while being reminded that every human being is created in God's image and is loved by God, regardless of one's physical and cognitive abilities. Such a reminder can provide the elderly and their relatives with a renewed sense of hope and purpose. It offers a way of measuring human worth and value that is often at odds with that of the secular world.

Rituals that are part of holiday celebrations and observances can also resonate with older people and their families. Connecting past to the present, such rituals weave together spiritual traditions with family experience and thus provide everyone with a sense of belonging to family, community and God. Not surprisingly, food is essential to most Jewish holiday celebrations, and almost every Jewish holiday has a particular food associated with it. The holiday treats served by facilities, or brought by families to their loved ones, can strengthen their sense of connection and belonging.[12]

---

10   Spiegel, Maria Cohn, "Old Symbols, New Rituals: Adapting Traditional Symbols, Ceremonies and Blessings". Ritualwell.org/lifecycles/primaryobject.2005-11-16.2926929096. Also, cf. Rabbi Cary Kozberg, "Let Your Heart Take Courage: A Ceremony for Entering a Nursing Home", *A Heart of Wisdom*, Susan Berrin, Editor, 1997: Jewish Lights Publishing.

11   The verses are Deuteronomy 6:4-8, and 11:13-21. Both passages contain the command, "Write (these words) on the doorposts of your house and on your gates."

12   Such holiday foods could include honey cake during the High Holidays, potato pancakes (*latkes*) during Hanukah, and *hamentashen* on Purim. Jewish/kosher bakeries sell these foods, and increasing numbers of supermarkets carry

When residential care facilities work to promote family celebrations of Shabbat and holidays, they contribute significantly to the spiritual/ emotional *healing* of each person in the family; this, in turn, helps them to better fulfill their mandate as caregiving organizations, as the following case illustrates:

In a meeting with the social worker during one of his monthly visits to his sister, Mr. S admitted the pain he felt each time he visited. He acknowledged his difficulty relating to his sister, whose dementia had progressed, and he grieved that their relationship had so vastly changed. Mr. S sadly described how his own life felt emptier as a result of this lost connection.

Knowing this family's history of religious involvement, the social worker encouraged Mr. S on his next visit to accompany his sister to the Sabbath worship service at the Home. A change occurred. Watching his sister's enthusiastic participation in the service, Mr. S remembered the meaning the service once had for his family and him in the past, a meaning that he re-experienced in the present. He realized that even with her cognitive limitations and declining capacity, his sister still manifested a strong spiritual side, as she continued to sing the songs that kept her connected to her religious and cultural roots.

Family members may experience many emotions – fear, frustration, grief, anger, guilt, exhaustion, embarrassment, isolation and abandonment – when witnessing their older relatives diminishing mental and/or physical health.[13] While moving a loved one into a residential care facility offers the opportunity of respite from hands-on care giving, relatives who visit daily and stay long hours, also risk exhausting themselves. Others may continue to experience the emotional toll of their past efforts, in addition to the current sadness they feel.

Since staff usually witness first-hand the difficulties family members may experience, they are often in a unique position to help families cope and find meaning of their experience. For those staff working with such issues, Jewish tradition can provide significant resources.

---

them as well.

13   Rabbi Deborah Pipe-Mazo, "The Psychodynamics of Caring for Aging Parents," Address and Person, *op. cit.*,p. 105. Also cf. Rabbi Cary Kozberg, *Honoring Broken Tablets: A Jewish Response to Dementia*, 2005: Jewish Lights Publishing.

Sacred Listening

The ever-present mandate to love our neighbors as ourselves calls us to listen carefully to the stories of another person's life and to do so with the knowledge that these stories have their own unique sanctity. Creating a safe space, offering a "listening presence" to family members who have been caregivers, allowing them to express their emotions and share their struggles without fear of being judged can all help promote acceptance and healing.[14]

As adult children understand their parent's life-journey, they can extend their own vision beyond the present situation to the value of their parent's life. This, in turn, can transform their experience of suffering into one of seeing the deeper purpose and meaning of their parent's life.

Members of the spiritual care staff, as well as nursing and other front-line professionals, can facilitate "family story time" – an opportunity for the older parent to tell his/her life story, and for the adult children to listen, receive and honor that story in order to help forge a deeper connection and mutual understanding. In this way, creating such a space is both an invaluable gift and also a holy act.

Dr. L, a 65-year-old successful physician with a thriving practice, was diagnosed with a rare debilitating neurological condition. He understood that his prognosis was poor. He endured much suffering over the four years he was ill, sometimes describing his situation as "falling off a mountain in slow motion."

During this critical and intense time, Dr. L and his family made a point of tending to some of their unfinished business. Given Dr. L's demanding professional life, his adult children had not been able to spend as much time with their father as they might have liked during their younger years. During his illness, Dr. L and his children chose to spend a lot of "quality time" together, and began to re-examine their relationship. In doing so, they were able to reconcile and repair their bonds with one another.

Dr. L availed himself of the opportunity to recreate and reconstruct himself into the kind of person he really – and finally – wanted to be. The experience also provided the family with the opportunity to reciprocate that love and to demonstrate their admiration for him in a way that, until the

---

14   Rabbi Dayle Friedman, "Help with the Hardest Mitzvah: Spiritually Supporting Family Caregivers," in *Jewish Visions for Aging,* 2008.Jewish Lights Publishing, p.78, figure 2.

illness, had not been possible. The illness also "forced" Dr. L. to be receptive to the care in a way that might not have been possible otherwise. This created a spiritual possibility for both the family and for Dr. L. and brought healing to both.[15]

When an older parent is no longer able to communicate, family members can still share stories and anecdotes with each other and with staff members. As their older relative hears the accounts, he/she will receive affirmation of the meaning of his/her own life and its influence upon others. In addition, another way of transmitting one's personal values and life lessons to one's family is through the creation of an ethical will, or spiritual legacy, often written in the form of a personal letter to one's dear ones, and reflecting an individual's beliefs and values to be passed on after his/her death.[16]

Judaism teaches that each human being is created *b'tselem Elohim*, (in the image of God). This can be particularly challenging in our culture, in which it is difficult to see any value or meaning in that which is frail and/or broken. Still, "brokenness" can be seen as an opportunity for creating a fuller whole, as the Hasidic master Rabbi Menahem Mendel Morgensztern (known as the Kotsker Rebbe) taught: "there is nothing more whole than a broken heart." Viewed in this way, "brokenness" – frailty, fragility and vulnerability – may be experienced by resident and family members as an opportunity for gaining wisdom and attaining healing, as the following poem, written by a daughter as she experienced her father's deterioration, attests:

As you aged, body connection became our major communicator.
It was difficult to watch you lose your memory.

One of my mirrors was gone, but like you I am learning to be in the moment
– not lacking history, but assuming it.

At some point I stopped reminding you that I was your daughter;
Our relationship had been transformed by your loss of memory:
We just were.

---

15   Naomi Mark, "A Perspective on Jewish Healing", in *The Mitzvah of Healing: An Anthology of Jewish Texts, Meditations, Essays, Personal Stories, and Rituals*, Person, Hara E. ed. URJ, p.37.

16   Cf. Josh Stanton and Hedy Peyser's chapter "Lessons of A Lifetime: Creating Ethical Wills In Senior Residential Care Settings."

Because of you I now understand that memory is most importantly about our bodies and our hearts; without these we cannot do justice to our histories.

You had a physical and emotional memory of justice and fundamental truth; You had an emotional essence; You were an essence in your stillness: You are the essence of Harry.

That's what I get: little fleeting moments of the essence of Harry.

It is a different way of seeing the world and I take it as a gift.[17]

Local synagogues and other Jewish communal and social service agencies may also provide additional support to residents and their families by providing regular visits to senior residential facilities, helping access community programs, or offering support groups and family counseling for caregivers, be they spouses or children. Staff who work with Jewish residents and their families should become familiar with such agencies as sources for additional information and support to Jewish families and their specific religious and/or cultural needs.

"From The Depths I Cried Out To You…":
Prayer And Ritual As Spiritual Resources

In moments of despair and uncertainty, prayer – whether expressed in the words of traditional prayer texts or in one's own spontaneous prayer – can be a powerful resource for hope and comfort for the caregiver who is experiencing emotional and spiritual distress.[18] Approximately 81% of caregivers for people with Alzheimer's Disease say they use prayer in coping with the demands of caregiving.[19]

Whether expressing heartfelt petitions, gratitude, or even frustration, prayer is a vehicle by which the caregiver can feel more connected to God – however "God" is understood – thereby putting his/her experience in a larger perspective. Some family members may have a practice of offering specific familiar prayers, or they may be open (and thus should be encouraged) to offer spontaneous prayer(s) from the heart. Others may find that simply meditating, and getting in touch with one's deepest feelings is helpful.

17   Gottlieb, A. *In Living Memory* (videotape), Toronto, Ontario, VTape: 1997.

18   Friedman, op. cit. p.79.

19   "Who Cares? Families Caring for Persons with Alzheimer's Disease," Alzheimer's Association, National Alliance for Caregiving. CD: 1999.

Creating prayer or meditation circles, particularly with a focus on healing, can be an important source of support for family members who are more spiritually inclined. Indeed, when a person offers a prayer or engages in other kinds of religious and/or spiritual experiences, they often feel comfort and healing:

I worried about my brother's health and well-being, as well as my own, because we were not taking care of our own bodies and spirits. In the face of long periods of helplessness, self-care seemed like the last item on our "To do" list. However, I did feel supported and deeply blessed that I had discovered the great treasures and teachings of the Torah some years before.

Reading and studying the Torah (the five books of Moses), learning and trying to understand what the rabbis and teachers of the past have said about its teachings, is an experience in which friends and I feel permission to discuss, challenge – even wrestle – with the texts. Using our heads and our hearts, we passionately seek where to find strength and meaning when the answers aren't clear. During such moments, I continue to learn that, despite the pain and exhaustion of this journey of caregiving, there can be openings, moments of profound intimacy and reconciliation which enable me to say it is a privilege.[20]

Sometimes the prayer is a poignant *cri de coeur*:

It is so painful, God, to watch my mother begin to falter.
I have always counted on her and now she needs to count on me.

I love my mother.
I can't stand the way our roles have reversed.
I don't want to see her in weakness.
I know this reversal is humiliating for her.
She doesn't want to feel helpless or dependent.
But she needs me now.

Help me God, to rise to this critical occasion.
Show me how to care for my mother with respect, tenderness and love.
Fill me with compassion and patience.

---

20   Susan J. Rosenthal, "Long Distance Caregiving for Elderly Parents", in *The Outstretched Arm*, Volume 4, Issue 1, Winter 2002-3/5763. National Center for Jewish Healing/JBFCS, www.ncjh.org.

Shield me from anger and resentment.
Calm my fears and give me strength, God.
Help me to seek out relief and support when the burden is great.
God, bless my mother with dignity and grace, with health and with
strength.[21]

While the challenges and accompanying responsibilities of caring for an older parent are indeed vast, they can be accompanied by wonderful spiritual opportunities. Within the complex and often emotionally-charged relationship of caregiver and care-recipient, the possibility of a new and stronger relationship – and partnership – may be created. In the face of vulnerability and mortality, when each longs to stay connected to the other, transcendence – with the support of staff, friends and community – can be achieved.

---

21   Rabbi Stephanie Dickstein, *With Sweetness from The Rock: A Jewish Spiritual Companion for Caregivers,* National Center for Jewish Healing, JBFCS, p.4.

Chapter 4
Judaism And Dementia[1]

Ellen Cahn, DHL

W hy do Jews tend to avoid discussing dementia as a personal issue? In the exploration of this topic, I would like to present contemporary thought, rabbinic teachings and theological issues that can challenge our conceptions of selfhood and relationship with God. I think dementia is scary for anyone to contemplate but is especially frightening for people who are focused on learning. "People of the Book" have a hard time facing the possibility of being unable to read. Harold Schulweis quotes Martin Buber, writing that he preferred books to people in his youth but changed his mind as he grew older: "I knew nothing of books when I came forth from the womb of my mother, and I shall die without books; I shall die with another human hand in my own" (Buber quoted in Schulweis 32).[2]

In order to discuss dementia, we have to face our own fears about its possible impact on our lives as a victim or caregiver. Tom Kitwood, a pioneer in the new thinking about dementia, admitted that there were several points in his own work when he considered giving up. He realized he had to confront his own fears about aging and dementia (5). I had the same issue when I was writing my dissertation on this topic. Acknowledgment of this apprehension is especially important for pastoral caregivers because we cannot be there for others in coping with their fears unless we can deal with our own. Our anxiety is increased by

---

1   This chapter is based on the author's doctoral dissertation, *When Our Strength Fails Us: Jewish Biomedical Considerations about Dementia*. Full details can be found in the list of references at the end of the chapter.

2   All references in parentheses can be found in the list of works cited at the end of this chapter.

living in what Stephen Post characterizes as a "hypercognitive" society that values intellectual and financial productivity and lowers the value of people who cannot meet this cultural expectation. He comments that "Descartes' *cogito sum* (sic) – 'I think, therefore I am' – is not easily replaced with 'I will, feel, and relate while disconnected by forgetfulness from my former self, but still, I am'" (*Moral Challenge* 5).

In this chapter I would like to explore the construction of an authentic Jewish identity that honors both our devotion to learning and recognizes the limits of cognition in religious experience and the definition of self. In doing so, I shall present rabbinic sources on Torah study. In terms of methodology, I think it is important to refer to individual experience rather than to just deal with abstractions; this approach is also recommended by Post as the starting place for ethical thought about dementia (*Moral Challenge* 13). There has been a paucity of patient and caregiver narratives by people who contextualize their experiences within a framework of Jewish identity compared to the volume of work written by Christians (including ordained clergy with Alzheimer's Disease, hereafter referred to as "AD") and people who do not state their religious belief, if any. Notable exceptions include the work of Morris Friedell, a person with dementia, and the articles about family experiences by Rachel Adler and Kim Chernin. Perhaps Jewish patients and caregivers may have a sense of shame in discussing a dementia diagnosis. Dr. M, a person with dementia (religion not specified) interviewed by Stephen Sabat, said: "Can it be that the term 'Alzheimer's' has a connotation similar to the 'Scarlet Letter' or the 'Black Plague'? Is it even more embarrassing than a sexual disease?" (29). Adler compares *tzaraat* (leprosy) and dementia in terms of stigma and states that "…hospitals and nursing homes in our culture are dwellings outside the camp." ("Those who turn away their faces: *Tzaraat* and Stigma", 154).

Our attitude toward dementia is important both in terms of bioethical policies regarding treatment options, allocation of scarce resources and end-of-life issues; it also impacts our role as pastoral caregivers. The answers to our questions about dementia may be at least partially determined by our phrasing of the questions. In the interest of fairness and to avoid marginalization, I think it is necessary to avoid pejorative language and labeling that result in the imposition of excess disability – a circumstance in which a person's poor functioning is caused or exacerbated by social attitudes rather than neuropathology. Malignant social psychology (Kitwood's term 14) focuses on a person's disabilities rather than recognizing his/her remaining abilities. Labeling also creates a distance between "us" and "them". This does not deny the existence of diagnostic criteria along the continuum of cognitive function, but recognizes the person with dementia as part of our community rather than totally "other." Christine Bryden and Morris Friedell, both people with dementia, use the analogy of the pointing of the bone, an Australian Aborigine ritual in which the sorcerer points a bone at the victim; the frightened person becomes sick and dies. They state "the manifestation of dementia is dependent on more than just brain pathology – our psychic resources, our social context and our spirituality are equally important." From this perspective, the authors argue that the trauma of diagnosis can be regarded as analogous to 'bone pointing' in Aboriginal culture. The impact of the diagnosis on the person and the people around him should not cause him to decompensate as the result of malignant social psychology.

I am using the term "person with dementia" rather than "demented person" in order to avoid making someone's disease his identity. This is the term used by DASNI (Dementia Advocacy Support Network International –http://www.dasninternational.org); their acronym is PWiD (rhymes with kid) in contrast to TAB (temporarily able brained). Post speaks of "...*deep forgetfulness*, a term I use to encourage compassion and solidarity..." (italics in original), although he also recognizes "... it is human development in reverse, an 'outliving of the brain', and an assault on human dignity." ("The Concept of Alzheimer Disease" 245). We can recognize the problems of this illness and at the same time not excessively valorize health. Cognitive ability is a value but not the only one.

It is encouraging to read the work of people with dementia who can speak for themselves. Friedell, who identifies himself as a liberal Jew, co-founded DASNI, which presents the voices of people with dementia rather than other people speaking for them. A person does not lose his identity or all cognitive powers the minute after receiving a dementia diagnosis, although a pattern of negative social interactions may be disabling as seen in an incident related by David Snowden of a man who was mute because "no one listens anymore" (195). A person's capacity to feel can continue long after he loses the capacity to speak. Furthermore, I use the term "person with dementia" because it affirms personhood, and thus implies that the person with dementia still has rights. Describing someone only as a dementia "patient" defines his core identity as an object in a hierarchal medical relationship. Such a description limits the exploration of his relationship with others and with God, by denying that he can still participate in the emotional and spiritual life of his community. A religious conception of personhood is also connected to the idea that every human being is created b'*tzelem Elohim* (in the divine image) – a status that cannot be forfeited even when a person's memories are erased.

Rabbinic Sources

The importance of Torah study, and by extension cognition, makes memory loss especially traumatic for Jews because learning is not only a religious requirement – it is also a form of worship. Louis Finkelstein's well-known aphorism notes that when he prays, he speaks with God; when he studies, God speaks to him. Studying connects a person with God, and thus the loss of this ability to learn can be seen as a diminution of the ability to serve and worship God with the mind as well as with the body. Neil Gillman asserts, "Judaism is the only religion in which study is equivalent to worship" (87).

Some of the rabbinic texts that address memory and forgetting with respect to Torah study are presented below, with the realization that no exact parallels correspond to the modern medicalized understanding of dementia.[3] The usable texts deal with forgetting rather than total helplessness, since in Talmudic times, people usually died of the diseases that constitute co-morbidity with AD, and vascular dementia before the full cognitive deterioration occurred. These stories do not furnish an exact paradigm for dementia because apparently learning was sometimes restored to the sages; a person with advanced Alzheimer's would be unable to relearn the teachings. While these passages do not address a modern PWiD's cognition, they do emphasize that the forgetful person must be treated with respect and that the victim is not always blamed for memory loss even at a time when the organic basis of memory was not understood.

---

3   All references to the Babylonian Talmud, Midrash Rabbah and the Zohar are from the Soncino translations unless otherwise specified. These texts and others are discussed in more detail in my dissertation. In Talmudic texts noted here, "b." denotes the Babylonian Talmud, followed by the name of the tractate (i.e.*Berakhot)*, which then followed by the folio page (i.e. 5b). In rabbinic texts, the abbreviation "R." denotes Rabbi or Rav.

Both effort and intention are important aspects of learning. *b. Berakhot* 5b has a statement by R. Yochanan to R. Elazar that the most important thing about Torah study is not how much the person learned, but whether it was done for the sake of Heaven. An extraordinary passage in *Midrash Rabbah* Song of Songs 5:21 stipulates heavenly reward for the effort regardless of the result. A pastoral implication is the merit of teaching Torah at a level commensurate with the ability of the person even if he/she may not be able to remember it for long.[4]

Emphasis on study is found not only in early rabbinic texts but also in the Zohar, the most influential book in Kabbalah (the Jewish mystical tradition), and also in Hasidic works. The Zohar asserts that the person who studies Torah will merit studying it in the world to come (Zohar 185a) and also states:

> It behooves a man to labor in the study of the Torah, to strive to make progress in it daily, so as thereby to fortify his soul and spirit: for when a man occupies himself in the study of the Torah, he becomes endowed with an additional and holy soul, as it is written: "the movement of living creatures", that is, a soul (nefesh) derived from the holy center called "living" (hayah). Not so is it with a man who does not occupy himself with a study of the Torah: such a man has no holy soul, and the heavenly holiness does not rest upon him. (Zohar 12b).

Some texts recognize disease as a cause of forgetting Torah, rather than moral turpitude or lack of diligent study. In *b. Nedarim* 41a, for example, we read about R. Joseph whose lost learning, which had been caused by illness, was restored by Abbaye, who reminded him of material that R. Joseph had taught previously. R. Joseph is again reminded of another teaching, in *b. Pesachim* 13a, by R. Ada b. Mattenah. When Rabbi (Judah ha-Nasi) fell sick and forgot his learning, R. Ḥiyya restored seven of his thirteen interpretations of a teaching from his learning and obtained the other six from someone who had heard Rabbi studying. (*b. Nedarim* 41a).

One of the most compassionate treatments of involuntary memory loss is related in *b. Berakhot* 8b and attributed to R. Joshua b. Levi:

---

4   For more on the continued importance of Torah study for the frail elderly, cf. David Glicksman's chapter "Torah Study in Senior Residential Care".

"...and be careful with the honor of an elderly scholar who has involuntarily forgotten his Torah learning, for we say that the second set of Tablets and the broken pieces of the first Tablets both rest in the Ark" (Artscroll edition). The same sentiment is expressed in *Menachot* 99a. Here R. Joseph, whose memory loss we read about in *b. Nedarim* 41b, exhorts his listeners not to be disrespectful toward a scholar experiencing memory loss that is not his fault and uses the same metaphor of broken tablets. We can think of the broken tablets as representing broken neuronal connections.

Theology

David Keck, a son of a person with dementia, refers to dementia as a theological disease: "Because this disease confronts us with our own radical finitude and with clear limitations of human powers, we have little choice but to turn to theology" (16). Dementia forces us to re-examine our theological beliefs and may be considered a return to chaos. Dementia, for Glenn D. Weaver, resembles the reversal of creation in the sense that the earth was created out of chaos; the mind of the AD sufferer descends into chaos (1986). He refers to the lament psalms especially Psalm 88 which makes specific reference to despair and alienation from God and other people.

Rabbi Dayle A. Friedman uses the metaphor of *midbar* (wilderness) and draws the analogy between the Israelite wandering in the unknown land of the wilderness and the experience of the person with dementia. She also speaks of the commandment to love the stranger. The person before us may not be the person we remember; he may also be a stranger to himself. Richard Taylor, another person with dementia, states: "There are times when I feel as if I am a stranger in a strange land, when the reality of the situation is that I am really myself in my own house" (150).

Another Jewish metaphor for dementia is Israel's exile from its own land in which the Jewish people were forcefully separated from the spiritual and quotidian lives they had known, yet were still able to maintain their community and belief system. The issue here is how a person can find meaning under vastly different circumstances including the transition from one's previous understanding of self. The nursing home may represent both metaphorical and physical exile. Kitwood notes "Dementia may be experienced as a form of bereavement: it means having to face two kinds of loss simultaneously – the loss of mental powers, and the loss of a familiar way of life" (29).

Dementia also forces us to examine the concept of theodicy because of the unfairness of this situation and the attempt to make it interpretable. Rachel Adler speaks of the difference between the suffering of the individual and the abstractions of the theologian who attempts to "uphold the perfect justice of the Eternal". She relates that her mother has not recognized her for two and a half years, yet turned to her twice and asked "why?" ("Feminist Judaism: Past and Future" 484). Regardless of our own beliefs about theodicy, this is a question that must constantly be addressed, even if it stirs up our own questions and doubts. In terms of pastoral counseling, it is important to note the warning of Jon C. Stuckey and Lisa P. Gwyther:

> Religion and spirituality are not panaceas for the dementia experience. Research has documented that the converse can be true. Religion, in particular, can become a barrier to emotional well-being because of unresolved anger toward God or some other divine force (Shah, Snow & Kunik, 2001). It is almost as if it is those who are overly dependent upon a strict doctrinal conception of God are those who are at the most risk for not being able to reconcile adverse events in their lives (295).

A PWiD's question about theodicy should be addressed with the same seriousness as a cancer patient's; we cannot assume that he does not know or understand what the issues are, especially in early dementia in which a person's sense of loss may be especially acute. Responding does not mean furnishing a definitive answer but acknowledging the person's pain. The person may be looking for assurance that this situation is not his fault or punishment. Believing that he is responsible for what has happened to him can cause excess disability as the result of the stress of feeling he is being punished and at risk for further punishment because he is angry with God. It is also important to view this belief not just as a theological question but as the result of existential terror. As Rabbi Elliot Dorff states:

> For the vast majority of people, however, you must translate the words to, "How do I cope with this?" or "How do I make sense out of this?" They may not be asking a question at all but simply using the words to express their agony, loneliness and fear. If you

respond to the questions with theological arguments, you will not be responding at all, for you have not really heard them(38).

In a different context, Rabbi David Greenstein speaks of faith as an attitude not as a belief. Dealing with theodicy calls for a theology of comfort rather than explanation (lecture, March 24, 2008).

What can Jewish spiritual caregivers offer? Religion can be both a coping mechanism and a source of connection linking the individual, God and faith community. In terms of coping, one aspect is stress reduction. Various authors have pointed out the role of spirituality and prayer in reducing stress in dementia and other illnesses for both for the person with the disease and the caregiver. Another closely related issue is the maintenance of selfhood. Bryden and Friedell point out the connection between spirituality and selfhood:

> We consider our spirituality to be important in maintaining personhood in dementia. In the face of declining cognition and increasing emotional sensitivity spirituality can flourish as an important source of identity. The self can be given meaning as a transcendent being beyond transient worldly difficulties of neurological impairment.

How can we empower people with dementia? There are several ways to do this. One method is simply listening. The person with dementia may experience grief over his/her loss over which he/she has the right to mourn. Listening to the person even if the words are repetitious is a form of validation because it recognizes that feelings matter. Authentically acknowledging a person's losses is conducive to trust; minimizing them can make the person feel that he is not being heard.

A second method of empowerment is what Rabbi Dayle Friedman calls the *mitzvah* model. Although she uses a sliding scale based on the person's abilities, a PWiD's ability to still perform a *mitzvah* (a commandment), however modified, is a way of maintaining self-esteem and a form of connection with God and the Jewish community. It affirms to that person that he still matters and is important to God.

A third method of empowerment is contextualizing the experience of PWiDs in Jewish terms. This would include helping attend and participate in religious services, however modified, in order to affirm that they are still spiritual beings. I remember one old man in synagogue who could still pray from memory, even though he was unsure about how to find his way home. To use a term from neurolinguistic programming, his presence in the worshipping community "anchored" the words and experience for him.

Music is also a powerful tool. A fellow congregant of mine remembered the melodies that she had learned in Hebrew school 70 years ago, but occasionally became totally disoriented in her own home and failed to recognize her husband. Rabbi Cary Kozberg comments that familiar traditional melodies work better with people with dementia ("Relating Gently and Wisely with the Cognitively Impaired" 351). He also notes that the traditional model of the rabbi has to be modified to reflect the ability to feel rather than the ability to understand (347).

The concepts of hope and consolation loom large in the Jewish historical experience, and certainly one way to offer hope and consolation is help those with dementia and their families to see the experience within the broader context of Jewish experience and imagery. Friedell states:

> Robert Davis was a Christian minister who wrote an inspiring book about his journey into Alzheimer's strengthened and comforted by Jesus' love. I'd like to match it from a liberal Jewish perspective. My equivalent of Jesus is the *Shekhinah*, the Indwelling Presence celebrated in the 23rd psalm. If I keep trying to do justice, to love kindness, and to seek intimacy with the *Shekhinah*, I can reasonably hope to experience the heartening and consolation that Davis did.

It is noteworthy that in Jewish tradition, the *Shekhinah* is not only understood to be the most accessible way of experiencing the Divine, but is also understood to accompany the Jews in exile, while also experiencing their pain.

To be sure, the hope and consolation that chaplains can offer is not the claim that the medical situation will miraculously change. Instead, it is the promise that, in spite of the cognitive loss, the person will continue to live as a spiritual being, that God will not forget or abandon his family, and that this promise will be a support to them as they cope. For caregivers, it may be the hope that God will give them strength, with a caution not to expect the impossible. In the language of the *Unetane tokef* (a well-known prayer recited on Rosh Hashanah and Yom Kippur), *teshuvah, tefilah* and *tzedakah* (repentance, prayer, and good works) can temper the severity of the decree, even if it cannot be annulled. People in the early stages of dementia can still attempt spiritual repair and reconciliation that can strengthen them for the hard times ahead.

The promise that God never forgets or abandons is a powerful message for persons with dementia, which becomes actualized when we create a "ministry of presence". In her analysis of pastoral presence with cognitively impaired people, Debbie Everett states: "In the midst of forgetfulness and the loss of control, the chaplain represents a God who never forgets us (Isaiah 49:15)" (86). In Jewish tradition, memory as an act of relationship with God is continually invoked liturgically. While we are exhorted to remember historical memories (e.g. the Exodus from Egypt), our requests of God to remember us are connected with existential concerns. During the High Holiday season between Rosh Hashanah and Yom Kippur, we ask God to *remember* us to life in at various places in the daily liturgy. The key issue is God's memory – not ours.

Works Cited

Adler, Rachel. "Feminist Judaism: Past and Future". *Cross Currents* 51:4 (2002).

– –. "Those Who Turn Away Their Faces: *Tzaraat* and Stigma" *in Healing and the Jewish Imagination; Spiritual and Practical Perspectives on Judaism and Health* ed. Rabbi William Cutter, PhD. Woodstock, VT: Jewish Lights Publishing, 2007.

Bryden, Christine and Morris Friedell. "Dementia Diagnosis – Pointing the Bone" (revision – May, 2001, slightly edited by Friedell in 2004) presented at the National Conference of the Alzheimer's Association Australia in Canberra, March, 2001. http://members.aol.com/MorrisFF/Bone.html accessed 6/16/08.

Cahn, Ellen Elisabeth. *When our Strength Fails Us: Jewish Biomedical Considerations about Dementia*. Diss. Jewish Theological Seminary, 2005. Ann Arbor, UMI, 2006. It can be ordered at http://disexpress.umi.com/dxweb.

Chernin, Kim. "Transcending Alzheimer's." *Tikkun* 18:4 (2003).31, 33, 66.

Dorff, Elliot N. "Rabbi, I'm Dying", *Conservative Judaism* 37: (4), 37-51.

Everett, Debbie. "Forget Me Not: The Spiritual Care of People with Alzheimer's Disease. *Spiritual Care for Persons with Dementia*. Ed. Larry VandeCreek. Binghamton, NY: the Haworth Pastoral Press, 1999.77-88.

Friedell, Morris. "I Want to Keep My Personality: A Jewish Journey

Through Alzheimer's". http://members.aol.com/MorrisFF/Personality.html. Accessed 6/17/08.

Friedman, Dayle A. "The *Mitzvah* Model: A Therapeutic Resource for the Institutionalized Aged". *The Journal of Aging and Judaism* 1:2 (1987).96-108.

– - "Seeking the Tzelem: Making Sense of Dementia". *Jewish Pastoral Care: A Practical Handbook from Traditional & Contemporary Sources* 2nded. Ed. Dayle A. Friedman. Woodstock, VT: Jewish Lights Publishing, 2005.

Gillman, Neil. *The Way into Encountering God in Judaism.* Woodstock, VT: Jewish Lights, 2000.

Greenstein, David. Zohar lecture March 24, 2008. Forest Hills Jewish Center, NYC.

Judaic Classics CD-ROM. Chicago: Institute for Computers in Jewish Life; Davka Corp and/or Judaica Press, 1991-2004. (Soncino Talmud, Midrash Rabbah and Zohar).

Kitwood, Tom. *Dementia Reconsidered: The Person Comes First.* Philadelphia: Open University Press, 2002.

Kozberg, Cary. *A Jewish Response to Dementia: Honoring Broken Tablets.* Woodstock, VT: Jewish Lights Publishing, 2005.

– -."Relating Gently and Wisely with the Cognitively Impaired". *Jewish Relational Care A-Z: We are Our Other's Keeper.* Ed. Jack H. Bloom. New York: Haworth Press, 2006.356.

Post, Stephen G. *The Moral Challenge of Alzheimer's Disease.* 2nd Ed. Baltimore, MD: Johns Hopkins, 2000.

– -. "The Concept of Alzheimer Disease in a Hypercognitive Society" *Concepts of Alzheimer Disease: Biological, Clinical and Cultural Perspectives.* Eds. Peter J. Whitehouse, Konrad Maurer and Jesse F. Ballenger. Baltimore: Johns Hopkins UP, 2000. 245-256.

Sabat, Stephen. "Surviving manifestations of selfhood in Alzheimer's Disease: a case study" *Dementia,* 1:1 (2002), 25-36).

Schulweis, Harold. "Coronary Connections: From a Hospital, Some Secrets of the Heart Revealed." *Jewish Insights on Death and Mourning.* Ed. Jack Riemer. New York: Schocken, 1995. 24-32.

Snowden, David. *Aging with Grace: What the Nun Study Teaches Us About Leading Longer, Healthier and More Meaningful Lives.* New York: Bantam, 2001.

Stuckey, Jon C. and Lisa P Gwyther. "Dementia, religion and spirituality". *Dementia* 2(3). 297.

Talmud Bavli: Tractate Berachos. Schottenstein edition. Vol 1.Brooklyn, NY: Mesorah (Artscroll),1997.

Taylor, Richard. *Alzheimer's from the Inside Out.* Baltimore: Health Professions Press, 2007.

Weaver, Glenn. "Senile Dementia and a Resurrection Theology". *Theology Today* 42.4(1986):444-456.

Chapter 5
Nurturing and Negotiating Holy Time in Foreign Spaces

Rabbi Sharon Mars

Judaism is a *religion of time* aiming at the *sanctification of time*.[1]

Jews live by a calendar which dictates that we reserve certain times of the year to connect with our people, our history, and indeed with time itself, our most precious commodity. In the course of the Jewish year, we celebrate times of rest (*Shabbat*/the Sabbath), miracles (*Hanukah*), and national redemption (Passover). We commemorate times of tragedy (*Tisha B'av*/the 9th of Av, Holocaust Remembrance Day) and of trial (Israel's Memorial Day). And we take time for contemplation of our deeds (*Rosh Hashanah, Yom Kippur*).

An older Jew may likely feel severed from the familiar and comforting regularity of the Jewish way of marking time after relocating from a private home into a residential care facility or other housing situation designed for older adults. In changing one's physical space – which is often accompanied by changes in one's personal physical condition – the new resident will face a whole host of complex transitions and challenges to his/her routine way of life. This is particularly true for Jewish residents who live in facilities under non-Jewish auspices.

---

1   All excerpts in this chapter are from Abraham Joshua Heschel's *The Sabbath, Its Meaning For Modern Man*, Meridian Books, The World Publishing Company, Cleveland and New York, and The Jewish Publication Society of America, Philadelphia, 1951; p.8. I am continuously inspired by his musings on holiness in time.

In my role as a chaplain serving Jews in hospitals and prisons, as well as senior residential care and hospice facilities, my challenge has been first and foremost to identify the needs of the residents in any of these facilities. Unless a city has a large Jewish population to support "Jewish" residential care venues (most frequently found in large metropolitan areas in the U.S.), more and more Jews will be living in facilities which do not primarily cater to the needs of Jews.[2]

There are times when, during the first or second visit with a new resident or patient, I come away with stories of lives lived sometimes in lands far away, sometimes in places familiar. Many of those lives have been lived under challenging circumstances. Some individuals can engage in life-review and describe in great detail their childhoods, marriages, child-rearing and golden years. Others may be largely unresponsive or uncommunicative, which is often the case with Alzheimer's and dementia residents. With that population, it is incumbent upon the chaplain to call or meet with their loved ones and caregivers to procure the puzzle pieces of their loved one's life. I meet some Jews who are constantly in conversation with the God of mercy and peace; others, plagued by doubt, feel no such divine comfort or nearness. Some have been anchored to synagogues their entire lives, while others have never been affiliated; some who search in earnest for the right moment to start the "conversation" with God, and others for whom the notion of God is not at all compelling or necessary in their spiritual lives. I have no necessary agenda when I enter a patient's or resident's room, other than to help that person feel more at home where s/he finds him/herself.

Despite the myriad manifestations of Jews I may encounter, the single common denominator I share with any Jewish resident or patient is the fact that we both identify as Jews. This fact serves to bind us together, most of the time opening the door to deeper discussion, more profound sharing of ideas, and an easier flow of communication regarding their needs and spiritual concerns. For example, while each Jew may understand and observe *Shabbat* (the Sabbath, or sacred day of rest) very differently, we often share a common reverence for the distinctiveness of that day. And so our lighting electric candles, sipping sweet grape juice and eating doughy *challah* (Sabbath bread) together ultimately

---

2   What I share in this chapter is based on my experience working in Columbus, Ohio, a mid-sized Midwestern city which has one senior care facility under Jewish auspices (Wexner Heritage Village).

constitutes an avenue to find other points of intersection in our Jewish lives. As simple as it seems, the sharing of these traditions and the telling of our stories can serve to bind us to our greater community, the Jewish people. They remind us that though we may be dispersed the world over, though our numbers may be greater or smaller in number depending on where we may be – the Jewish calendar is a part of all of our lives, helping us to make the time we have to live more meaningful by making it more sacred.

Labor Is A Craft, But Perfect Rest Is An Art[3]

But what of a Jewish resident who lives in a facility which is not primarily focused on serving the needs of Jews? For the Jewish resident who seeks to find connection with his/her tradition, living in a non-Jewish facility can be profoundly isolating. Sometimes the only Jewish connection a person may have is his/her family, but family alone may not always be able to fulfill the person's religious/cultural needs. The responsibility then falls to the group of professionals who are responsible for caring for that person.

After I make initial assessment of a person's spiritual needs, my role as chaplain is to contact the various team members who work in the facility. Connecting with them is essential to establishing the parameters for helping the Jewish resident/patient achieve his/her spiritual or religious goals. A good collaborative relationship between the Jewish chaplain and the non-Jewish staff is important in maximizing the quality and quantity of Jewish engagement which will most likely revolve around the holy days which dot the Jewish calendar. This requires striking a delicate balance of time, provision of resources, in-service learning opportunities, and consistent maintenance to ensure that staff feels adequately supported and equipped to address to the special wants and needs of the Jewish members of their care communities.

Ideally, a facility's administration and staff will expressly support these efforts. I have found that it is best to start by introducing oneself to the head administrator(s) and other chaplain(s) if any are on staff. Initial discussions should include identifying goals (e.g. Jewish residents should be notified in a timely manner as to any Jewish holiday activities), and clarifying values (e.g. Jewish residents should be treated in a way which honors the fact that all human beings were created in the divine

---

3   Heschel, p.14.

image). Once a preliminary conversation has taken place, it is helpful for the Jewish chaplain to be introduced by the administration to the rest of the staff – social workers, activities specialists, nurses and aides – to determine a strategy to involve the entire team in carrying out the stated goals of how caring for the needs of the Jewish population can be met.

Reality to us is thinghood, consisting of substances that occupy space; even God is conceived by most of us as a thing.[4]

Engendering sensitivity to Jewish sacred time among non-Jewish staff members can be complex and multifaceted. An orientation or in-service educational opportunity can be useful in introducing staff to important religious concepts and practices, which should address such questions as:

"What is 'keeping kosher'?"
"Why won't Mrs. Goldstein eat a cheeseburger?"
"Why does Mr. Shapiro want to hang a boxed scroll (mezuzah) on his doorpost?"

Central to all of this, however, is the subject of sacred time. Among other questions that should be of interest are those that ask:

"Why won't Mr. Shapiro eat bread during Passover?"
"Why does Mrs. Goldstein insist on getting her hair done every Friday before sunset as opposed to Saturday morning?"

As noted above by Heschel, the spiritual antidote for "thinghood" is repossessing and redefining the meaning of time. Jewish time is distinguished by phases of *ḥol* (ordinary or mundane time) and *kodesh* (holy time). Thus, when candles are lit every Friday before sunset and *Shabbat*/the Sabbath begins, time changes from being "ordinary" to being "holy" and sacred. It is no longer that which we try to "kill", nor is it a commodity which we cannot seem to expand enough to fill in with the "busy-ness" of our lives. *Shabbat* and the other holidays of the Jewish calendar transforms time into that hallowed series of hours

---

4   Ibid., p.5.

and minutes within which we can refresh and renew ourselves. With each and every home- and synagogue-centered holiday, Jews gather to remember who they are, praise their Creator, and actualize the divine commandments which guide and give meaning to life.

Not A Date But An Atmosphere[5]

Indeed, there is much for staff members in non-Jewish facilities to learn about caring for Jewish residents. It often necessitates their learning an entirely new Jewish lexicon, filled with foreign or little-understood Jewish concepts, and possibly stepping outside of one's comfort zone in order to occupy another's. For example, it is crucial to communicate the significance of *Shabbat*/the Sabbath to staff. Occurring weekly, *Shabbat* not only dominates the Jewish consciousness, but also the calendar itself. Jews who observe *Shabbat* also spend time preparing for it. Thus, Fridays should feel different for Jewish residents; time and effort can be spent in preparation, with special care taken to tidy and clean common areas of the facility. Other subtle changes can also symbolize the approach of *Shabbat*: *challah* can be sold in the gift shop; the beauty and barber shops might be busier; families may be encouraged to visit, and Jewish preschoolers may entertain the residents. Staff should know how to respond to "*Goot Shabbes*" or "*Shabbat Shalom*" – traditional Sabbath greetings to which one would reply by repeating the phrase with a smile. Additionally, observant Jews may ask non-Jewish staff to carry out tasks from which they themselves are prohibited by Jewish law on *Shabbat*, such as pushing elevator buttons or using electricity.

Administrators may consider creating learning incentives for staff, enticing them with extra vacation time or CEU credits for going that extra mile in creatively and consciously making the facility a more hospitable place for its Jewish residents. Staff should continually be encouraged to attend workshops on topics as varied as "The Special Needs of Holocaust Survivors," "Making *Shabbat* a Day of Rest," and "Useful Russian and Yiddish Phrases". Obtaining this kind of knowledge about one's residents can be empowering for nurses and aides, as well as for social workers and administrators. Ideally, one result might be staff taking the initiative to create Jewish holiday programs – doing arts and crafts activities, forming committees, organizing a range of activities, offering learning opportunities about Judaism for other residents, in

---

5   Ibid., p.21.

consultation with Jewish residents and the chaplain. Ultimately, an atmosphere of *yiddishkeit* (Jewishness) can be created, infusing the staff with a sense of pride and the residents with a feeling of truly being at home.

Creating "A Palace In Time"[6]

Any educational efforts that promote a higher awareness of Jewish needs will have a tremendous impact on creating a sense of harmony among staff members and Jewish residents in non-Jewish extended care facilities. Moreover, it will enable those Jewish residents to create "a palace in time," as Heschel teaches, a place where they can encounter God, each other, and their own selves. In this way, they will experience the guidance, nurturance, clarity of purpose, and peace they so deserve, so that this time of their lives will truly be sacred.

Postscript

Since the publication of the first edition of this book, I have created a program which seeks to further enhance the religious and spiritual lives of Jewish residents in non-Jewish extended care facilities. I function as the Jewish Community Chaplain of my community. Limited in time and resources, and finding it difficult to fully serve the needs of unaffiliated Jews by myself, I initiated a volunteer project matching Jewish residents in various local senior care facilities with Jewish volunteers. Asking the local rabbis to each nominate one or two notable *tzedek-* (justice) minded individuals from their congregations, I found a dozen energetic and eager souls ready to perform the commandment of *bikkur cholim* (visiting the sick) in the community. Over a six-hour training course (over two separate evenings,) they learned and bonded as a group to become para-chaplains in what is now the Nadav Spiritual Volunteer program.[7] In addition to the initial training, volunteers continue learning at monthly group gatherings to add to their Jewish pastoral care knowledge and refine skills.

The most important part of the program, however, is the actual visitation between the para-chaplain volunteer and resident. The goal is to foster long-term relationships which are enhanced by significant spiritual conversations and experiences between Jewish para-chaplains

---

6   Ibid., p.15.

7   "*Nadav*" is Hebrew for to donate, to volunteer.

and the Jewish residents who live in non-Jewish senior residential care facilities. Volunteers are strongly encouraged to develop strong bonds with staff members by connecting them to Jewish resources, building bridges between the residents' families and their respective facilities, and simply being another set of "eyes and ears" to assist staff in the daily care of the residents. Each resident visited by a Nadav Spiritual Volunteer is automatically part of the Nadav Network, a system I developed to make sure that, should a resident's physical condition change and/or is hospitalized, he/she doesn't "fall between the cracks". By way of a small framed sign posted in the resident's room, the facility is reminded to call the rabbi (i.e. myself) if and when this resident has a change of condition or location. Once contacted, I alert the Nadav Spiritual Volunteer assigned to that resident, so that either one of us (or both of us) may respond as needed – whether it be making a hospital visit, reciting the *vidui* (final confession) or simply praying with the resident. For a Jewish resident who may otherwise feel disconnected from his/her community, a friendly face from that community showing up often to visit goes a long way in telling the person that the connection is there … and it still matters.

Chapter 6
Jewish Spiritual Care in Senior Residential Settings: A Nurse's Perspective

Deaconess Linda Frank, BSN, CTS

The challenge we face when we aim to provide exceptional care to our elders living in long-term care settings is that the activities and services which make our residences superior are those for which an organization cannot be reimbursed. For instance, we know that increasing the nursing staff-to-resident ratios improves the quality of care a resident receives, but we do not receive increased dollars in reimbursement when we increase the number of nursing personnel assigned to care for a resident population.

This is also the case when it comes to the spiritual care we would like to include in senior residential care facilities. The value of spiritual care, in any medical venue, seems to be difficult to measure, and an historical lack of quantifiable evidence of spiritual care's value stymies efforts to include a full array of spiritual care services in an organization's budget or in a health care manager's reimbursement. With the exception of the laudable hospice benefit requiring the inclusion of a spiritual care provider as a core member of the interdisciplinary team, health care insurance programs generally lack such provision or requirement.

Yet it is widely accepted that illness and aging prompt spiritual or existential reflection; the questions which surface with advancing years can be sources of spiritual distress for anyone. It stands to reason, then, that our care of the sick and elderly is incomplete, perhaps ineffective, when the spiritual needs of our clients are not identified and addressed. Despite medical advances and the expertise of counseling services, the absence of comprehensive spiritual care limits the effectiveness of a resident's interdisciplinary care team. That is, without the anecdotal and experiential evidence provided by spiritual care services, the care team works with incomplete data. This chapter will discuss the benefits of faith-specific spiritual care, and offer anecdotal evidence of the benefits to having a rabbi or Jewish chaplain on the staff of senior residential care facilities which are home to Jewish residents.[1]

Treating The Whole Person

Holistic health care is the goal of the many health care practitioners who advocate for the inclusion of spiritual care providers on the team of professionals of senior care facilities. These advocates embrace the philosophy that wellness entails all aspects of a patient's self, integrating physical, emotional and spiritual components. This philosophy insists that we be as attentive to a patient's emotional and existential distresses as we are to their physical illnesses. Doing so allows us to provide them an opportunity to live in a state of maximum well-being.

My perspective on this issue is unique. I worked as a Registered Nurse for thirty years before changing careers. Now I am employed as the Christian chaplain for a Jewish health care campus. Working alongside two rabbis, I provide spiritual care to the Christian hospice clients and residents of the campus's residential and rehabilitation facility. It was as a nurse providing care to our older and terminally ill populations that I recognized the spiritual care void that exists for some; now as a chaplain I have seen the anecdotal evidence attesting to the value of faith-specific spiritual services.

My contribution to the broader discussion of Jewish spiritual care in a senior residential care setting is to share my experiences and observations as well as related comments from my colleagues. Individuals come to mind whose stories represent the emotional and spiritual healing that timely faith-specific spiritual intervention provides our elder population and their families. I remember the family of a Jewish man to whose bedside I as the hospice chaplain-on-duty was called. The patient's daughter was expecting me, and stood at the doorway to her father's room. She smiled and politely thanked me for coming, but her body was positioned to prevent me from entering the room. I asked if there was anything I could do for her or for the family, to which she responded carefully, "We would prefer someone who speaks Hebrew."

---

1   It goes without saying that the same would be true for non-Jewish residents, regardless of the nature of their care facility.

What a gracious way to state her family's desire for a visit from a rabbi! Such frank and honest requests from families and residents are not common. Most of us are not comfortably forthright at such a time – all the more reason to note the significance of the daughter's words to me. Significant life events and milestones often elicit a need or desire for attention and care from our particular faith's leaders or representatives. Some of these occasions can be anticipated, such as a person's death (especially if it's anticipated, as it often is in a senior residential care setting). But there are also spiritual needs or situations which we cannot foresee, and others about which we would remain unaware without the guidance of a spiritual care specialist.

One senior residential care resident's situation illustrates this point: I was asked to visit a Christian woman with a long history of paranoia and depression whose manipulative behaviors had recently escalated. A social worker was involved in her care and a psychologist had visited with her more than once. Although the resident was being treated pharmacologically, she still continued to lash out at family and triangulate staff. In addition, she continued to isolate herself, leaving her room only for meals. The cause of this woman's increased anger and fearful behaviors was attributed to her recent move into the facility. I was asked to meet with her, in part, because other attempts to help her were unsuccessful.

My conversation with this woman began slowly. We talked about her adjustment to her new living arrangements and her frustration and anger regarding her loss of independence. I respected the silences which punctuated our conversation and after one such pause she mentioned that a teenage niece was recently baptized. Another pause was followed by a confession: "I was baptized when I was a teenager. I did it because all my friends were being baptized," she said. *"I was baptized for the wrong reason."*

I knew the particular significance of baptism in this woman's Protestant denomination, so I immediately understood her anguish. Peer pressure is not a valid reason to participate in a public sacred ritual intended to proclaim one's religious fidelity and commitment. This resident's revived memory left her feeling ashamed at the very least, and at worst caused her to question the current state of her relationship with God.

I knew my response needed to be both knowledgeable and respectful of the teachings of this woman's church. Conversation and prayer, rooted in her denomination's language and precepts, eventually enabled her to feel reconciled with God despite her childhood misstep. The following day I found my client cheerful, walking outside her room, on her way to attend a resident activity program. To be sure, her paranoid and manipulative behaviors never disappeared, but she maintained a trust that she was loved by God.

Although this story's details are Christian, its lesson informs spiritual caregivers of all faiths. While chaplains are trained to identify spiritual distress and provide spiritual comfort to persons of every faith, there are occasions of spiritual crisis when the attention of faith-specific pastoral care is essential in healing spiritual pain. Such attention can be offered authentically only when the chaplain has intimate knowledge of both the overt teachings and the nuances of a particular tradition. For Jewish residents of a senior residential care facility, it is more than beneficial to have a rabbi or Jewish chaplain on staff. Indeed, if it is the intent of the facility to provide its residents with complete and timely holistic care – it is *necessary*.

"Holistic care," one nurse asserts, "is the most compelling reason" to have a rabbi available to visit with Jewish residents and their families, and to teach the nursing care staff who care for Jewish families. This nurse observed that visits from the rabbi offer her residents and their loved ones "comfort, support and understanding" at critical or stressful moments, such as at the time of a Jewish resident's death. Like the daughter who declined my pastoral visit by requesting prayers spoken in Hebrew, we all are inclined to turn to the traditions of our particular faith in times of crisis. We find solace, encouragement and strength in the prayers, traditions and faith language unique to our spiritual heritage. This is true regardless of the degree with which we have been connected to a congregation or participated in the activities and rituals of our faith. In the senior residential care setting, Jewish residents and their family members are consoled and supported by the familiar sound of a Hebrew prayer. Even persons who describe themselves as "not religious" appreciate the Jewish chaplain's compassionate presence and his/her advice and counsel regarding their faith's rituals and tradition.

The staff benefits, too.

Personal anecdote: "I'm not a religious person," a daughter confessed to me at the time of her mother's death, "but my mother was. Can you tell me what I can do now to honor her faith?" My experience with Jewish practices at the time of death enabled me to answer this daughter's question for the moment; and I, with the daughter's permission, communicated her request to our rabbi who then guided her through her mother's funeral and shiva (the seven-day period of mourning).

It is not only Jewish residents and their loved ones who benefit from the supportive presence of a rabbi or Jewish chaplain at the time of a resident's health crisis or death. The nurses and other staff members benefit as well: with the presence of the chaplain, they are free to concentrate on their clinical and clerical duties for the welfare of the other residents in their charge. They can offer the family their condolences without needing to be the family's primary source of emotional support. Indeed, they are appreciative of the chaplain's intervention when emotional outbursts of grief or anger demand counseling skills beyond their expertise. Moreover, nursing staff members will at times seek personal consolation from the rabbi. In other circumstances, the rabbi's presence with the family permits nursing staff members to step away from the situation for a moment when they need to acknowledge their personal feelings of loss related to the resident's passing.

While the rabbi interacts with residents and families, attentive and interested staff members are learning about Judaism. They observe how to respond respectfully in the first moments after a resident's death by lighting a candle in the room, opening a window, covering reflective surfaces. Some staff members may have questions before attending a Jewish funeral or making a *shiva* call to a family in mourning. Moreover, when the rabbi has an ongoing presence with staff, residents and families, there are multiple opportunities for him/her to provide anticipatory teaching. For example, when the rabbi learns that a member of a resident's family is a *kohein* (a descendant of Aaron the High Priest), the rabbi can explain to the staff why this relative will not enter the resident's room once the resident is actively dying or when the resident is deceased.[2]

When staff is caring for someone who is an Orthodox Jew, the rabbi can guide the staff's interactions with family members, explaining, for instance, why male visitors will avoid shaking hands with female staff persons. Such education helps the nursing staff honor the resident's

---

2   Part of the code of conduct delineated for the Aaronic family entails that they do not come into contact with dead bodies. Cf. Leviticus 21.

and family's religious practices, and of equal importance, it protects residents and their loved ones from awkward moments with staff who might otherwise misinterpret behaviors that are unfamiliar to them.

Thus, one of the most important roles of the rabbi or Jewish chaplain in a senior residential care facility with a Jewish population is that of teacher. Assuming that a facility's employees want to provide residents with competent holistic care, we can rightly believe they are open to, perhaps even hungry for, as much information as possible about the cultural and religious practices of their residents whose faith is different from their own. As a member of the caregiving team, the chaplain does more than provide spiritual support to Jewish clients and answer staff questions as they arise; he/she also educates about Judaism in more formal settings, beginning with orientation for new employees. In our facility, the rabbi is introduced to new employees and presents general information about Judaism and the particularities around caring for elderly Jewish persons. Involving the rabbi in staff orientation gives the message to employees that the organization's commitment to holistic care for all residents is rooted in a religious and spiritual commitment to a Higher Purpose. In addition, new employees' meeting the rabbi during the orientation process establishes a relationship which welcomes staff to consult with him/her if or when questions/concerns should surface in the future as they care for their Jewish residents.

Educational in-service sessions led by the rabbi are beneficial particularly before major Jewish holidays. The purpose of these sessions is to teach staff about the origins, significance and traditions of each approaching holiday, so the staff can honor the religious practices of Jewish residents, and also be sensitive and alert to the emotions that a holiday may elicit. Due to staff turnover, it's important that this type of in-service training be offered on a regular basis for all new employees for every holiday. Although the subject matter would remain fairly constant, there should always be time for questions, based on individuals' experiences, or responding to unique issues affecting residents.

Additional learning opportunities can also be useful to nursing staff. In-services covering a variety of subjects such as the Jewish dietary laws, the observance of the Jewish Sabbath (*Shabbat*), common Jewish phrases, and the beliefs and customs of Orthodox Judaism can help make staff more sensitive to the religious and cultural backgrounds of residents and thus enhance the level of cultural diversity and sensitivity. In addition, some employees may enjoy spending time with the Jewish chaplain in Scripture study. Our experience with this program has been that its success depends on when it is scheduled (usually at a time that coincides with the staff's meal break), and more importantly, how informal and open the learning atmosphere is to various attitudes and interpretations.

Spiritual Assistance For Residents And Families

When appropriate, the rabbis/chaplains should attend regularly scheduled residents' care-planning meetings. While discussing a plan for the resident's care, the chaplain, the resident, and the family establish a relationship, and the chaplain gains insight into their religious beliefs. Joining with nurses, social workers, and family members, he/she will provide important information which can affect a resident's care. In addition, the chaplain becomes a trusted advisor for the resident and family, and acts as a liaison between them and the medical team.

When the resident experiences significant health changes or crisis, the chaplain interprets plan-of-care options to the family, especially if they involve matters of Jewish law, custom, or practice. Familiar with the medical issues and terminology, the rabbi can help explain in layman's terms the nature of each treatment option; he/she can address the family's understanding of issues such as life support, tube feedings, Do-Not-Resuscitate orders, and hospice services. For persons who are connected to a congregation, the chaplain can facilitate the inclusion of their rabbi in the decision-making process; and for families who are not affiliated with a local synagogue the chaplain may become their spiritual advisor. With dual expertise, the facility's Jewish chaplain bridges medical and religious worlds so that a family's decisions are both informed and faithful.

As a teacher, advisor, and guide, the rabbi/chaplain provides attention, support, and education which are appreciated and valued by both families and nursing staff. As one nurse reported, "I have watched the rabbi work miracles". "Your supportive presence and advice during our time of crisis and grief will never be forgotten," wrote one son in a note to a facility's rabbi. "The rabbi has been more than a teacher to me," one Christian nurse commented with intense admiration, "he has been my role model."

The Jewish chaplain who is well integrated into a facility's caregiving staff displays more than supportive behaviors, religious and spiritual expertise and a gift for teaching in a variety of settings. He/

she becomes an emissary and exemplar of the Jewish faith. Through effective mentoring and teaching, the chaplain models a principled lifestyle which values the worth of every person, responds to every situation with compassionate loving-kindness and is respectful and non-judgmental, even in challenging circumstances.

It is likely that in a Jewish-sponsored senior residential care center most of the nursing staff will not be Jewish themselves. Nevertheless, through their relationship with the Jewish chaplain, caregivers can discover and affirm a common understanding of the divine call and life's purpose. Their close working relationship, as I have observed, inspires and encourages those who share a personal goal to integrate the tenets of their faith into their daily living habits. Working with the Jewish chaplain, they can find spiritual meaning in their work.

Conclusion

Faith-specific spiritual care is an essential component of comprehensive and holistic elder care. While every human being has a spiritual or existential perspective on the meaning of life, suffering and joy, and death, not everyone is religious nor does everyone align with a religion or faith community. The Jewish community itself reflects this spiritual diversity. In the senior residential care setting that is home to Jewish residents, a rabbi or Jewish chaplain holds a vital role, guiding, advising and teaching the Jewish families he/she meets, enabling the nursing staff and others on a resident's interdisciplinary team to provide holistic care, to assist residents and their families through difficult decision-making processes, and support them during the last days of a resident's life.

Chapter 7
The Ethics Committee As A Venue For Pastoral Care

Rabbi James R. Michaels

People familiar with ethics committees in acute care facilities know that they play an integral role in the care of people in the last stages of life. Such committees meet at least weekly to discuss issues which are immediately pressing: questions of medical futility; allocation of limited medical resources when the demand is greater than the supply; unpleasant and difficult decisions about a patient's care when relatives are unable or disagree about what that treatment should be.

As Nancy Berlinger, a noted specialist in medical ethics at the Hastings Institute, has observed, ethics committees in long-term care facilities have less-defined roles. The issues presented usually do not involve discontinuation of care, and often residents' wishes are well known. Instead, long-term care ethics committees may be drawn in the direction of counseling with family-members as they accompany their elderly loved ones on their last journey.

One of the dimensions of my role as chaplain at the Charles E. Smith Life Communities is to serve as staff liaison to the ethics committee. Over the years, I have seen how the committee can play a different and integral role in the care of our residents. Since most of our decisions are not imminent ones concerning life or death, we can assume a role more oriented toward pastoral care. This chapter will examine various scenarios in which such a role is appropriate.

History Of The Ethics Committee Of The Hebrew Home Of Greater Washington[1]

Until the mid-1970s, issues of medical ethics were rarely discussed by individuals. What changed at that time was the awareness that medical technology could keep patients alive, but not necessarily guarantee any quality of life. Cases like that of Karen Quinlan made Jews focus attention on issues which previously had been theoretical points of Jewish law. Jews wanted to know if they could sign advance directives and living wills, and what they could request in those documents.

As the only Jewish health care facility in the Washington DC area, the Hebrew Home became the natural location for discussion of these questions. Even though its ethics committee was already well established, it was reorganized to respond to community needs. Although empowered to decide on cases, the committee's meetings usually took an educational format. Local rabbis and doctors sat on the committee. They researched questions of ethics and presented papers for discussion. The meetings were primarily held in the evening hours, in order to accommodate members of the community who were interested.

Later, as members of the community became more aware of their options with regard to making health-care decisions, the format was changed again. Official meetings were held once each quarter. A mechanism was also developed to create case consultation committees; requiring only a few members of the committee, these could be convened at short notice, sometimes within a few hours. It has been within these case consultations that the pastoral role of the committee has been most clearly in evidence, as the following cases will illustrate.

Caring For Residents

Mr. and Mrs. C, an elderly couple from South America, were admitted to the facility's sub-acute rehabilitation unit. Both husband and wife had recently been brought to the United States and did not speak any English. Mr. C was in hospice care, and his wife was quite frail.

---

1   In 2006, the name of our facility was changed to the Charles E. Smith Life Communities, but which it had been known as the Hebrew Home since its founding in 1910. I am indebted to my predecessor, Rabbi Seymour Panitz, for information in this section of the chapter. The first full-time chaplain of the Hebrew Home, he was witness to the formation of many aspects of our mission. I wish him and his wife Barbara many more years of life and good health.

She was eventually transferred to one of our long-term care units. A problem presented itself when the woman, still in control of her cognitive abilities, was asked if she would sign a "Do Not Resuscitate" (DNR) order. Her children had lived in the United States for a long time, and understood the importance of leaving such instructions.

Mrs. C initially said she did not want to sign the DNR form. According to her children, she had said that she did not want to give up on any medical care to keep her alive. Her doctors had recommended against administering CPR in the event of a heart attack because it could result in pain and suffering due to broken ribs.

The couple's children asked for a consultation with the ethics committee. They told the committee that while they respected their mother's wishes, they also feared that she did not understand the implications of not signing a DNR. They wanted to know what they could do. The consultation committee explained that because the resident was cognitively intact, they could not unilaterally change her wishes without her consent. However, it was recommended that the mother be brought to talk with the committee members in the hopes that they could persuade her to sign the form.

A few days later, the family brought Mrs. C to visit her husband. By coincidence, they passed me in the hall and introduced me to their mother. They explained that I was "a Jewish minister". As she was an Evangelical Christian, meeting a member of the clergy carried significant importance for her. By additional coincidence, two members of the initial consultation committee were nearby; we quickly convened a second meeting, and sat with the woman and her family.

I explained to Mrs. C (through her children's translation) that her desire to live was admirable, but that if she elected to receive CPR, it could result in significant pain and suffering. I asked her to consider if she wanted to live with such pain. She thought for a few minutes, and then said, "I will now leave everything in the hands of God." She agreed to sign the DNR.

Mr. C died a few days later. Mrs. C lived for another four months and passed away quietly with her family nearby.

The pastoral implications of this case were significant. First, even though the children had expressed respect for their mother's choices, there may have been some subliminal conflict between them and her. Second, by using a chaplain's "priestly authority", I was able to overcome Mrs. C's resistance to considering what might be in her best interest. Third, once she agreed to sign the DNR, she had peace of mind and was able to enjoy the remainder of her life with her family.

Care For Medical Professionals

As a large skilled-nursing facility, the Hebrew Home is able to have a number of physicians on staff. Although residents are permitted to maintain their own personal physicians, most take advantage of the services of the staff doctors. I was surprised one day when one doctor asked if he and his colleagues could learn more about the Jewish perspective on end-of-life issues.

He explained that, over the years, they had been told Orthodox Judaism insists that end-stage patients be kept alive at all costs. They were distressed because they thought patients' best interests were not being served. They also perceived a wide gulf between the beliefs of Orthodox and non-Orthodox Jews in this area. I invited the doctors to attend the next quarterly meeting, and said I would arrange for an Orthodox rabbi to attend.

I called Rabbi Yitzchak Breitowitz, a noted expert in Jewish medical ethics and a professor of law at the University of Maryland. An Orthodox rabbi, he had previously been a member of the ethics committee, so he agreed to attend the meeting.

Rabbi Breitowitz explained that Jewish law's views on this subject are much more subtle than normally assumed. He said that most people are familiar with *responsa* (rabbinic answers to questions of Jewish law) in English stressing the commonly known position which discourages withdrawal or withholding of life support. There are others in Hebrew, he said, which present options for withholding life support. He said, "We're obligated to preserve life, but we're also obligated to prevent suffering." He indicated, therefore, that this issue is much more subtle and nuanced, even among Orthodox Jews.

The immediate result of this meeting was that doctors were reassured when they discussed this. They felt more comfortable discussing hospice care with families of Orthodox residents. After hearing Rabbi Breitowitz, the doctors felt more comfortable referring their non-Orthodox Jewish patients who believed they had no choice in end-of-life matters, to rabbinical authorities for consultation.

There were other positive results. The doctors realized that Jewish law is not radically at odds with their own beliefs. Non-Jews felt they were not forced to adhere to a specific approach to end-of-life issues; Jews felt more comfortable with their own tradition.

When Religious Tenets Guide A Decision

As medical technology becomes increasingly adept at keeping people alive, the nuances of Jewish law expressed by Rabbi Breitowitz have become important for how chaplains and other staff deal with end-of-life issues. The two examples offered below illustrate how these nuances – or their absence – can affect ethical decisions and thereby influence a resident's quality of life.

The first example, which occurred in another SRC, involved Mrs. G, who had spent a long time in a hospital in New York, before being moved to the Jewish long-term care facility in a different city where her daughter and son-in-law, an Orthodox rabbi, were living. Mrs. G had a number of co-morbidities and it was the opinion of the facility's medical director that additional medical interventions would probably have no positive effect for Mrs. G, and might actually shorten her life.

A meeting was convened between the daughter and her husband, and members of the staff, including the medical director, the social worker, and the chaplain. The medical director explained Mrs. G's condition to her daughter and son-in-law, and suggested that the best course of action would be to keep her as comfortable as possible at the nursing home rather than send her to the hospital. The social worker then told them that the plan was to move Mrs. G to a part of the building that would better assure her comfort. Expressing respect for the family's traditional beliefs, the chaplain gently introduced the possibility of hospice services, adding that many of the Jewish chaplains who work in hospice are themselves Orthodox rabbis. Using language that he knew they would understand, he told them that the nursing home staff were indeed partners with God in caring for residents, including Mrs. G, but that given the realities of Mrs. G's situation, God might be saying that it was time for us human beings to step aside, and let Him take over.

As the chaplain spoke, both the daughter and son-in-law nodded their heads, and then expressed their deep appreciation for all that was being done for Mrs. G. They explained, however, that they of course could not "give up" on Mrs. G and would do everything they could to preserve her life. In addition, they would continue to consult with their own rabbi, who lived out of the city, but who was Mrs. G's rabbinic "power of attorney". They would share the conversation with him, and would abide by his decision as to how they should proceed.

Ultimately, the family decided to follow a more aggressive, rather than palliative, course of action. A day or so later, at the insistence of her daughter, Mrs. G was sent to the ICU "for tests". When the chaplain went to visit her in the hospital he saw that Mrs. G had a feeding tube, and that she had been placed on a ventilator. She did not respond visibly to any verbal stimuli. During the chaplain's several visits, Mrs. G's daughter and her sister who had come in from out of town, expressed appreciation for his visits and the prayers that were being offered for their mother. Mrs. G remained in the ICU for three weeks until she died.

The postscript to this case is that after Mrs. G's death, the chaplain spoke with another Orthodox rabbi in town in whose congregation Mrs. G's daughter and son-in-law are members. The chaplain raised the case with this rabbi. To be sure, in order to respect both the family's privacy and HIPAA regulations, no names were used. The rabbi, however, was very aware of the situation firsthand. When the chaplain asked the rabbi's opinion about the family's decision, his answer was "there are some *rabbanim* (rabbis) who are more *machmir* (strict) in these situations, and others who are not." He explained that his inclination was to follow rabbinic authorities who are more sensitive to the bigger picture and the nuances involved. He added that, if they had approached him, his religious counsel to the family would have been very different.[2]

For some, the above case would argue that a religiously conservative approach will not be sufficiently sensitive to the resident/patient's situation and quality of life. However, another case in which I was personally involved, demonstrates that such a religiously conservative approach can at times arrive at a correct – and effective – decision.

Mr. T, a resident in his late 80s, had lived in the skilled nursing facility for several years; his wife still lived independently. Upon her husband's admission, she had told the staff that he had been active in his synagogue and wanted to attend our services as often as possible. We made arrangements for volunteers to bring him almost every day. Even though he had significant dementia, he still enjoyed his time spent in religious services.

As the years passed, the man's physical condition worsened and he came much less often to the synagogue. Eventually it was determined that he needed dialysis three times each week to survive. The family was in a quandary. He had never signed an advance directive, nor had he ever told anyone in the family if he wanted to extend his life. Together with social workers and me, the family engaged in a long discussion

---

2   From a personal conversation with Rabbi Cary Kozberg.

about what to do. Would he have wanted to continue his life, albeit with dementia? The family had difficulty making the decision. Some said that as a religious man, he would want to prolong his life. Others felt he was too pragmatic and wouldn't want to live with dementia and ill health.

Finally, one of the nurses treating the patient mentioned that he had a permanent IV port inserted in his arm. On the basis of that fact, the family came to the conclusion that he would want to prolong his life. They began sending him for dialysis treatments three times a week. On the days when he didn't go, he would be brought to services. Although he had trouble focusing on the prayer book, he enjoyed hearing the words of prayer and even made up some of his own. When called for an *aliyah*,[3] he would recite the words loudly and clearly. Moreover, he enjoyed spending time with his family and friends, as well as residents and staff in the nursing facility.

In this case, the religious impulse to "preserve life" prevailed, with the result that the patient continued to have a modicum of quality in his life. The family felt gratified that they could continue to visit, share music, and occasionally go to services with him.[4]

Pastoral Care For Nursing Staff

Even though physicians are responsible for residents' medical care, the nursing staff is more involved in the day-to-day decisions and care. Because of their close contact with residents, nurses can experience strong feelings of care and concern for the patients in their charge. This usually results in great dedication to their work. When they feel a patient's best interests are not being met, these same emotions can lead to frustration. At such times, they may need strong statements of support for their work and for their concern. The following case, involving conflict between nurses and a family member, will illustrate how the ethics committee can provide this important affirmation.

Mrs. B was an immigrant from the Philippines, in her nineties,

---

3   Literally "to go up." An *aliyah* refers to the honor of being called to say the blessings before and after a part of the Torah is read during a worship service.

4   Some situations present even more difficult dilemmas for Jewish chaplains, particularly with regard to role-definition. Cf. Ephraim Karp, "Ethical Considerations in Chaplaincy" *National Association of Jewish Chaplains Newsletter*, Kislev 5771/December 2010.

greatly debilitated, and able only to speak a native dialect. Although many of the staff members speak Spanish, they were unable to communicate with the resident; instead, her granddaughter assumed the responsibility for communicating and translating for the staff. Even though Mrs. B's sons had medical power of attorney, the granddaughter (whose mother was deceased) was more involved in decisions about day-to-day care. She visited almost every day, while the sons came usually only once each week.

Over time, the granddaughter became very intrusive in the resident's care issues. She demanded that nurses respond immediately to her wishes, often accusing them of neglecting her grandmother. For example, she insisted that the resident be turned frequently while in bed, or weighed almost daily. The nurses were distressed, wanting to care for the woman, but also anxious not to be pulled away from caring for other residents by the granddaughter's demands.

The unit's nurse manager came to me, nearly in tears because of the situation. She said her staff was unable to function properly. She pointed out that objective criteria, such as the absence of bed sores and maintenance of body weight, indicated that Mrs. B had not been neglected. The granddaughter, however, would not desist in her demands, even when shown the data.

A case consultation was organized; Mrs. B's sons were asked to attend. The granddaughter also came, bringing her own senior-care advocate. After all the data were presented and all parties were allowed to present their concerns, the advocate told the granddaughter that she was not acting in her grandmother's best interests. The committee told the sons that they should become more involved in their mother's care.

The case consult had affirmed the nurses' care for Mrs. B as well as the other residents on the unit. Word about the decision quickly spread among the facility's nursing staff. They realized the ethics committee was indeed a forum where they could express their concerns and find needed support when they were facing difficult issues of caregiving; nurse managers from every unit now attend all quarterly meetings.

Issues Affecting Holocaust Survivors And Their Families

As Paula David writes elsewhere in this book,[5] Holocaust survivors

---

5   Cf. her chapter "More Battles: Age-Related Challenges for Holocaust

in residential care facilities often relive many of the traumas they experienced in their younger years. In our facility, we've occasionally encountered issues that affect such residents, along with members of their families and staff entrusted with their care.

One memorable case involved Mrs. A, a woman who had survived the Nazis' attempts to wipe out the Jews during World War II. She had immigrated to the United States, married and had a family. Now in her late 80s she was admitted to our facility for rehabilitation after a heart attack. Since she had an increased risk of further cardiac events, her daughter was asked if she as medical power of attorney wanted to sign a DNR order. The daughter adamantly refused, claiming that since her mother had survived the Holocaust, she wasn't going to give up in the face of death.

Mrs. A's nurse manager and other staff felt that the daughter was not aware of the ramifications of her decision. They requested an ethics consult, at which time the case was thoroughly discussed. I was asked to speak to Mrs. A's daughter. At that meeting, she and I reviewed all the issues of her mother's case. She once again stated her opposition to signing a DNR form. I explained that while we all respected her right not to sign the form, it was important that she understand that, because of her mother's frail condition, application of cardio-resuscitation could result in cracked ribs, from which she would endure great pain. I asked if she was willing to commit her mother to the possibility of suffering without any chance of relief. After a couple of days, the daughter agreed to sign the DNR form. Fortunately, the mother was discharged before any additional events occurred.

Since many of the nurses in our skilled nursing facility come from Third World countries, many know little or nothing about the Holocaust. At one meeting of the committee, some of them asked for more information about the events of that horrible time, and how they have affected not only the survivors but also their families. An adult child of a survivor was invited to speak to the subsequent meeting. He explained how he and his fellow "children of survivors" had learned to deal with the post-traumatic stress experienced by their parents, including issues of survivor's guilt, the trauma of remembering the witnessing of repeated beatings and public executions, and the lasting effects of malnutrition.

The nurses were very grateful for the information the man

Survivors".

presented. However, one committee member realized that much more education was needed, and that one of the world's great resources – the United States Holocaust Memorial – was nearby and readily available. Tapping monies available in a fund for staff education, the facility organized a trip for 22 nurses, representing each nursing unit and coming from a wide variety of countries-of-origin, to the Memorial. A special docent was assigned to the group, which made its way through the various exhibits with careful intention. Witnessing the photographs and graphic description of the persecutions, forced deportation, and dying (or living) in the concentration camps, the caregivers expressed greater sensitivity to what residents in their care had experienced.

Summary

In addition to offering guidance and advice, ethics committees have the opportunity and the power to provide pastoral care for residents, family members, and staff. Unlike their counterparts in acute-care settings, these committees do not need to make major commitments of time and energy to participate. To the contrary, the experience at the Hebrew Home here in Washington indicates that quarterly meetings are sufficient for the committee's work; of course, there should be a mechanism for quick consultations.

Family members and staff should be notified and reminded frequently and regularly of the availability of the ethics committee for consultation. In addition, we have found it important that *all* staff, including GNAs and support staff, understand that anyone can come to the committee if he/she feels a resident's interests are not being served. While it may occasionally be necessary for the committee to impose a decision if disputing parties do not agree among themselves, meetings of the ethics committee should stress mediation, allowing those concerned to formulate a workable decision.

Finally, promoting a pastoral response to ethical issues sends the message that disputes in patient care need not result in irreconcilable anger and hurt feelings. Instead, ethics committees in Jewish residential care facilities can demonstrate how Jewish principles and values can help to resolve such issues and, in the process, establish a model of *kedushah/* sanctity for the entire community.

Chapter 8
Revealing The Jewish Voice In Clinical Pastoral Education

Rabbi Sara Paasche-Orlow

There is a long tradition of Jewish communal responsibility for elders and every major Jewish community has a clear social service mechanism to care for the poor elderly. With the "extreme aged" (85-105) compromising the fastest growing segment of the population and the Baby Boomer generation beginning to enter their later years, one of the pressing questions we face today is: how will we tend to the physical and spiritual needs of older adults, their families, and caregivers as people live longer with more medical acuity, more loss of physical independence and a high incidence of dementia?

Clinical Pastoral Education (CPE) is a model for the training for chaplains that involves group learning, group supervision, clinical work, individual supervision, writing *verbatim* and theological reflection. Originating in the Protestant tradition but now embraced by all faith traditions, CPE is the dominant mode for training chaplains in the United States and has transformed chaplaincy by providing professional certification for a field that was formerly an underdeveloped element of clergy training. To become a certified chaplain, students must successfully complete four units of CPE training. A CPE student working full-time can expect certification to take two years to complete (one year with four units of CPE, plus an additional year of working after CPE).

Prior to establishing our CPE program, it was evident that our residents at the Hebrew Rehabilitation Center had pastoral care needs far beyond what a two-person Religious Services department could provide. As I began to consider how we might expand the role of chaplaincy at HRC, it became evident that there was a demand for more chaplaincy training in Boston and a local and national need for Jewish chaplaincy training programs. With the full support of the HRC administration in 2006 we began the only Jewish Geriatric CPE training site then accredited by The Association for Clinical Pastoral Education (ACPE). Our program is grant funded, predominantly by local Jewish foundations and individuals. As of Spring 2011, it has provided training for 52 students, eleven of whom have completed multiple units.

From the program's inception, we were blessed to have the gracious assistance of Reverend Mary Martha Thiel, an exceptionally gifted chaplaincy supervisor in the ACPE community with a longstanding professional commitment to interfaith chaplaincy. Her excitement, skill and commitment to fully exploring and realizing the contextualization of CPE in a Jewish healthcare institution have been essential to the creation of this program. The learning and experiences expressed in the following pages reflect an interfaith journey that we have been on together.

What follows will describe some of the features of providing pastoral care to residents in senior care living venues: longer term relationships, life reflection, end-of-life care, and dementia care. In addition, some of the key features of how traditional CPE training has been adapted to reflect Jewish values, theology, and cultural norms in a geriatric setting will also be described.

Caring For Our Seniors: Hiddur P'nei Zaken

Pastoral care in a senior care environment is different from hospital chaplaincy in many ways. However, the most dramatic difference is the length of time the chaplain can spend with a given resident. In contrast to the brief time which a hospital chaplain has with a patient (sometimes just one visit), chaplains in senior residential care facilities may have months, even years, of opportunity for relationship building. Many residents in these facilities may have outlived their friends and family and are alone in the world. For others, the spouse or children might also need support and guidance along the way. Geriatric pastoral care involves building relationships, being part of an interdisciplinary care team that cares for the whole person by providing spiritual support and at times religious guidance, in the face of the inevitable decline and episodic catastrophes that can accompany the aging process.

When people feel that their days are numbered, they often reflect on the meaning of their lives, and try to find ways to cope with the suffering and sorrow they experience. Jewish memories and cultural identity can provide ways to help Jewish residents continue to find spiritual meaning and fulfillment at this time in their lives. To be sure, how people approach and express "religion and religiosity" can vary greatly. Reflecting the demographics of the American Jewish community, the vast majority of Jewish residents in senior care centers are not Orthodox. In addition, most are Jews from birth. As such, their membership in the Jewish community is not contingent on religious practice or even belief in God. They are Jews by simple reason of birth. Yet, even without a religious connection to their Jewish identity, many may have a strong cultural desire to stay connected with other Jews, and wish to live in a recognizably Jewish atmosphere where they feel "grounded". In such an atmosphere, Jewish residents may not only desire to reconnect culturally, but they may also to seek Jewish ways of engaging with existential issues.

For example, I remember one day, during his first week at HRC, a man came to my office in his wheel chair. He had lived his whole life with cerebral palsy and said to me, "There is not much more I can do with my body, but I want to work on my *neshama*" (soul). He was able to articulate what others know deep down but often need help articulating. Part of Jewish chaplaincy training is learning to meet Jewish individuals "where they are" Jewishly-speaking, and to respond to their desires to make life meaningful and worth living *in Jewish ways*. Some of the people with whom I've worked have lived for years with debilitating conditions, yet seek to create a life that is meaningful and fulfilling. They want to use their time and their abilities for reflection, emotional and spiritual development, and fulfillment of goals and dreams. The Jewish chaplain can help facilitate nurturing Jewish identity by helping them to draw on the strength of lifelong Jewish memories. It is these memories that can inspire them to better integrate a sense of hope, love, forgiveness and purpose into their souls.

In addition, chaplains in senior residential care facilities play an important role on palliative and hospice care teams. When death is imminent, residents, their families and the care team itself can all benefit from what the chaplain can offer in the way of pastoral care. A chaplain can provide support in helping a family transition from medically aggressive goals for their loved ones to ones that stress palliative care. Such situations may present both theological and pastoral challenges from a Jewish perspective, because in Jewish medical ethics there is a tension between a firm commitment to saving life because it is God-given, and the acceptance that death is also a part of life. A family may have spent decades advocating for the best possible treatment for a parent or spouse, and thus may find it difficult to go in the direction of palliative care when it becomes evident that curative measures are no longer relevant. Some families might choose the more aggressive approach until the end, even though it may appear to outsiders that their loved one will continue to suffer. In addition, sometimes it is difficult to discern if the decision that is made reflects the patient's value system, or that of the family, or is a response by the family made out of desperation. On the other hand, some families may believe that for all intents and purposes their loved one's life is over, and thus, seem almost eager to allow the person to die. In situations like these, a Jewish chaplain can be invaluable in helping both the family and care team determine appropriate goals for care in a culturally and religiously sensitive way.

Another unique aspect of end-of-life care particularly in Jewish senior care venues is working with survivors of the Holocaust and their families. As time passes, the population of Holocaust survivors is dwindling rapidly. At our facility, survivors make up approximately 2% of the resident population, and in the next several years, we can expect to lose all of them – and there will only be their memories to cherish and keep alive.

One survivor, Rebecca, confided to me when she was dying that throughout her life, as she lay down to sleep, she would recite the names of the six siblings she had lost to a death camp. As she approached her own death, she was full of guilt that she had been the one to live – and soon she would be facing them. She was also saddened that with her death, their memory would die as well. To add to her distress, she had chosen to forego a difficult amputation – a choice which made her dying sooner more likely. Choosing against having the amputation made her feel that she was choosing to die. She was wracked with guilt. In order to care for her, the entire team became involved in helping her find resolution, feel loved, and assure her that her memories would live on after she was gone. With so much care and concern surrounding her, she was able to die peacefully.

Working with individuals who are coping with dementia is also a significant part of chaplaincy in senior care facilities. Caring for this population means staying connected to "normal" reality, while realigning oneself to their reality in order to offer moments of reassurance and love. Jews with dementia who have lost their cognitive abilities still have a lifetime of Jewish memories and experiences. For these individuals, hearing a Jewish melody, being greeted with a traditional greeting like "*Gut Shabbos*" (Good Sabbath, a traditional Sabbath greeting) on a Friday afternoon, can often evoke strong and wonderful memories of times when the person felt the loving presence of family and community all around him/her. Often Jewish residents who are non-verbal may still be able to recite long-known prayers and chant verses from the Torah quite easily because these were learned during their childhood years.

In order for chaplains to be fully present to, and fully effective for the people with whom they work, they must be aware of and understand the agendas and baggage that they themselves may bring to the work of pastoral care. Jewish chaplains in particular need to be educated about the range of choices within the context of Jewish medical ethics, know how to access ritual, text and prayer resources, and be theologically grounded so that they may authentically accompany residents and families in their journeys. On a daily basis, chaplains who work in senior care settings witness many small joys and acts of loving-kindness. At the same time, they also bear witness to a lot of suffering and death. Thus, because they too are human, they must learn the self-care needed to be able to come into these environments and enter these relationships with an open heart. These are among the goals of Jewish CPE education.

Jewish Clinical Pastoral Education[1]

Jewish CPE training requires a partial reconstruction of the historically Protestant framework of CPE, to form a program that is guided by Jewish learning, culture, and theology. There are core theological concepts in CPE training that may need to be understood differently or even transformed in Jewish contexts, such as *vocation, forgiveness, faith, hope,* and *eternal life.* Specific process aspects of CPE that may also need "tweaking" include aspects of language, group prayer, group process, individual supervision, and cultural competence. Jewish chaplains certainly benefit from training that is rooted in their

---

1   I want to express my gratitude to Reverend Mary Martha Thiel, my colleague in beginning our program, an inspiring CPE supervisor, and *hevrutah* partner (study partner) in thinking through all these issues.

own Jewish religious and cultural tradition, and prepares them to serve Jewish patients with very different spiritual, cultural and religious needs from those of many Christian patients.[2]

From Vocation To Mitzvah

The Christian religious notion of vocation or "calling" has historically been an important concept in CPE as chaplaincy students develop their sense of religious identity, spiritual path, and future professional focus. While Jews may not use the phrase "being called", nevertheless the concept of performing *mitzvot*, (commandments), is based on the understanding that at Sinai, God "called" the Jewish people – individually and collectively – to engage in these specific behaviors as a way of imitating God's holiness and making it accessible in the world.[3] For many Jews, the concept of *mitzvah*/commandment is a more fitting paradigm than that of a personal "calling". To be sure, while the phenomenon of God's calling an individual is very present in the prophetic tradition, the concept of vocation still *sounds* somewhat foreign to some Jewish ears. However, the sages of the Talmud did teach

---

2   Editor's note: Rabbi Paasche-Orlow describes one aspect of a growing trend in Jewish religious life – the desire to provide professional pastoral training for rabbis, cantors, and laity who work in health-care settings. As she notes, the historically Protestant Christian nature of this training has undergone significant changes. In large measure this is due to the growing number of CPE programs which are distinctively Jewish (such as at Hebrew Rehabilitation Center) as well as the availability of books and resources which help non-Jewish supervisors (i.e. those who provide the training) understand the Jewish dynamics of this field. Having instituted a similar training site at the Charles E. Smith Life Communities in Rockville MD, I can attest that such programs add much to the spiritual care available to residents, family and staff. Trainees are able to visit more residents than one full-time chaplain, and the aura of pastoral presence is extended much more strongly throughout the entire facility. While this chapter describes one method of CPE training, there are other approaches to learning this discipline. Individuals interested becoming clinically-trained chaplains, as well as administrators interested in creating CPE programs in their facilities, should explore all the options. Information can be obtained from the Association of Clinical Pastoral Education (www.acpe.edu) and the College of Pastoral Supervisors and Psychotherapists (www.cpsp.org) – JM.

3   Cf. Exodus 19: 5-6 and Leviticus 19:2. For more on the concept of holiness in Jewish tradition, see Cary Kozberg's chapter, "You Shall Be Holy: The Roles of the Jewish Chaplain in Senior Residential Care Settings".

a similar idea: through sacred acts of *g'milut chasadim* (loving-kindness), individuals could become close to God by imitating divine attributes.[4] In addition, engaging in daily *talmud Torah* (study of Torah and sacred texts)[5] and daily prayer, are the ways by which a person can connect with God. The phrase "holding fast to Torah" means to remain true to the values of Jewish tradition, including continuing the work that previous generations of Jews have done to help other Jews: creating and supporting immigrant aid societies, *bikkur cholim* (visiting the sick), caring for Jewish communities internationally, supporting Israel, and fighting for social justice. Orthodox Jewish teaching affirms that to hold fast to Torah, Jews must observe traditional *halakhah* (Jewish law) and that this is God's clear command to all Jews. To be sure, there certainly are Christian theologians who express similar ideals.[6]

Yet another similarity to the notion of "being called" is a teaching of the sages about the purpose of work. They understood work – human labor – as a fulfillment of God's will. They noted that just as we are commanded to rest on the Sabbath as a way of experiencing the sanctity of time, so we should understand that the productive efforts we put forth during the work week are also sacred; from the laws prohibiting certain kinds of work on the Sabbath, we learn what kinds of work *must* be done during the week.[7]

Forgiveness And Teshuva

Another central tenet of chaplaincy as understood from a Christian perspective is forgiveness – understood to mean that people make peace with themselves, with others, and with God. From this perspective, God's grace and forgiveness often override God's justice ("Forgive us our sins as we forgive those who sin against us"). Human sinfulness is understood to be universal and related to the phenomenon of Original Sin, which is removed through the suffering and death of Jesus. Faith in the redemptive meaning of the Passion is the way to experience

---

4   Babylonian Talmud, Sotah 14a.

5   For more on the importance of this activity, cf. David Glicksman's chapter, "Torah Study in Senior Residential Care".

6   Cf. Frederick Buechner, *Wishful Thinking: A Theological ABC:*, "The place God calls you to is the place where your deep gladness and the world's deep hunger meet."

7   Irving Greenberg, *The Jewish Way*, 1988, New York, pp. 134-135.

God's forgiveness. Thus, it is believed that a prayer to God can evoke forgiveness, regardless of how the offended party responds.

In the Jewish tradition, the concept of forgiveness has historically been understood differently. In biblical Israel, there was an annual Temple ritual that ritually made for a spiritual cleansing of the people. In addition, individuals were expected to correct their wrongdoings, change their ways, and "do *teshuvah*" (engage in acts of repentance). This included making amends with those whom one had wronged and asking forgiveness of God as well. To be sure, while pardon from God might be assured, pardon from offended parties would come only when the offended parties forgave their offenders.

After the Temple was destroyed in the year 70 CE, the ritual of atoning sacrifices were replaced with prayers offered in the synagogue. Three times a day, a worshiper recites a prayer to God for forgiveness. The weekday morning service includes a special section of supplication (*tachanun*) which amplifies this. Sinning, repentance and forgiveness is based on the assumption that God has given human beings free will. An essential part of the Jewish understanding of sin and human accountability to God is the affirmation of free will as a gift from God.

In addition, the liturgy and rituals of the High Holidays, culminating in Yom Kippur, the Day of Atonement, are a modern version of this ancient Temple atonement ritual. During the month of Elul, and in the days between Rosh Hashanah and Yom Kippur, Jews are encouraged to engage in *teshuvah* – to repent and return to the right path of goodness before humanity and God. The liturgy of the High Holiday service centers on the concept of forgiveness. Indeed, a key prayer of Yom Kippur is the *vidui* (confession), and a version of it is traditionally said when death is approaching. Whether in its traditional Hebrew form or in modern renditions, the final *vidui* provides a person the opportunity to "finish one's business" – to let go of old grievances, to make peace with others, with one's self and with God.

Faith And Skepticism

One requirement of some CPE programs is the writing of essays in which students discuss their "Experience of Faith". Jewish CPE students will likely express their experiences in different terms from their Christian colleagues, because the concept of "faith" is understood differently in Judaism.

A central theological tenet of Judaism is not just "believing in

God" but rather *trusting* God. Because this trust is based on God's redemptive deeds on behalf of the people of Israel, it is not a "blind" faith or trust. At the same time, when Jews engage in learning Torah – trying to understand God's word and God's will – discussion and asking questions is encouraged, even expected. The name by which the Jewish people are known – "Israel" – means "one who wrestles with God". In modern times, this teaching has encouraged modern Jews to express their connection with the Divine, not necessarily by confessing their faith, but by questioning, and wrestling with it. Thus, Jews rarely *declare* their personal faith. Indeed, a rabbinic student may go through years of seminary without ever articulating his/her faith directly. But it unlikely that he/she will finish without having struggled with it.

Associated with the call to fulfill God's commandments are the biblical words, *na'aseh v'nish'mah* (we will do and then hear.) These words express the idea that the Jewish response to God's call is to *act* – rather than just "have faith". Through actions – doing the commandments – we try to hear God's voice, or feel a certainty of God's presence. It is true that many Jews believe that "works" alone are important, and "faith" remains an afterthought, that "acting Godly" is more important than believing in God. Although it may be challenging to Jewish CPE students to have to articulate their experiences with "faith", nevertheless, it is still an important part of their preparation for pastoral care work. Thus, with such divergent starting points, discussions of faith should be approached with sufficient knowledge and sensitivity to the significant differences between Christianity and Judaism. Similarly, Christian clergy should also know that while Jewish patients may identify strongly as Jews, they may not be at all fluent in the "language of faith".

Tikvah And Tikkun Olam

It is to be expected that a program rooted in a Christian theological perspective, would include ongoing references to Jesus. Although such references are meant to call forth the blessings of love and hope, these references will be foreign, perhaps alienating, to almost all Jews because of whom the referent is. To be sure, many Jews, including some rabbis and rabbinical students, often have a superficial understanding about the role of Jesus in Christian faith.

Similarly, Christians often are not aware of Jewish teachings about hope, and how Judaism understands the future as a time of the ultimate physical and spiritual redemption of humanity ("the messianic age"), and or how the concept of *tikkun olam*, repairing/healing the world in connected to realizing this vision. These teachings often form a Jew's religious or cultural understanding of hope and the purpose of life, and thus are important for chaplains to understand. To be sure, the conviction that humans can repair the world, and that the future holds the promise of a world healed and redeemed are concepts not necessarily affirmed by all Jews. There are Jews who eschew this theology, and see no evidence that humanity is progressing or that the world is improving. Thus, they certainly are not prepared to accept that the Messiah has already come. Nevertheless, they continue to live their lives wanting to make the world a better place and do so by donating time and resources to help others, support the State of Israel and/or work for various social justice causes. Though they may not believe that world is improving, they still feel called to ease some of its suffering however they can, and work for a better future for coming generations. This may be particularly true of those individuals who survived the Holocaust.

The Rewards Of Heaven

Set forth in traditional prayers, and rabbinic lore, Jewish teaching affirms a life after this one – a world-to-come. Based on the belief that we human beings are accountable to the Sovereign of Sovereigns, the dominant teaching by the sages of the Talmud is that notions of afterlife are tied into the notion of reward and punishment, which will occur in one fashion or another in this world, or the next.

However, it is also true that many Jews do not resonate with this concept. The reason may have to do with the fact that to the average Jew, a belief in an afterlife, – "going to Heaven/Hell" – is so entwined with Christian belief and theology. Consequently, belief in an afterlife may not be on a Jew's theological radar screen, and therefore Jewish pastoral care at the end of life may look quite different from that offered by Christian pastoral caregivers. Jews who do not believe in a life after this world often hold that the lasting impact of their deeds and their progeny is the vehicle by which they will transcend death. For them, the focus is on living righteously and ethically in this life, with an eye to leaving a legacy for future generations – not for the sake of a heavenly reward but for the continuation of the Jewish people, and because it is the right thing to do.

Language

Again, because CPE's roots are planted in Christian "soil", it is understandable that the traditional CPE learning process will use language that is specifically Christian. Terms like "didactics", "devotions", and "ministry", for example, are ubiquitous, but may be unfamiliar to Jewish CPE students. Changing uniquely Christian terms to words that are either neutral or have a Jewish connotation, can certainly further a sense of trust and engagement. For example, changing the term "didactics" to *limudim* (Hebrew for "study") can set a tone of Jewish relevance and a sense that the learning experienced in CPE is part of a greater endeavor to uncover God's will in the world. Another accommodation might include the use of relevant Hebrew and Yiddish terms. When used to promote more affective responses, these can help Jewish students to explore their own ideas and feelings in a deeper and more personal way. Additionally, translating terms like "devotions" and "ministry" to *avodah* gives the connotation of worship and sacred work. Learning in a CPE program designed specifically with a Jewish framework opens possibilities for self discovery and reflection that Jewish students may not experience in other CPE programs. However, all programs can strive to be more inclusive of Jewish perspectives and experience.

Prayer And Worship

Many CPE training programs begin their sessions with prayer, and encourage participants to share their own spontaneous prayers. Jewish CPE students may be accustomed to beginning their day by praying some form of the traditional morning service *(shacharit)*. Yet, if these students come from various religious backgrounds and theological outlooks, organizing such a service in which everyone can comfortably participate may present challenges. Orthodox Jews may have their concerns (i.e. blessings should not be recited if the time and circumstance is not appropriate) and more liberal Jews may have their particular concerns (i.e. masculine language should not be used exclusively in referring to God). Spending a few moments to reflect on a text, meditate, or sing may suffice to begin a session on a spiritual note, although always with sensitivity to the group's diversity.

It should also be noted that while the modality of spontaneous prayer – "sharing a prayer" – is a common part of Christian spiritual life, it has traditionally not been a focus of the Jewish worship experience. Liturgical prayer is dominant in Jewish life, and there are certain times when personal prayers are invited. For example, when the prayer

Shma koleinu ("Hear our voice") is recited during the silent *Amidah* prayer,[8] the individual is invited and encouraged to insert personal words and requests. Another opportunity for offering a private personal supplication is at the time of lighting the Shabbat candles, just before Shabbat begins.

It should be noted, however, that in recent years more Jews have begun to include elements of spontaneous prayer in various contexts. Still, some who wish to pray may find it difficult to do so with sincere devotion (*kavanah*), and may experience spontaneous prayer as somewhat foreign, even inauthentic. For this reason, CPE within a Jewish context should include opportunities for Jewish students to explore the meaning of prayer, how they relate to prayer, their relationship to prayer, in order to learn how to utilize prayer as a component of offering pastoral care and creating a pastoral relationship in ways that feel authentic.[9]

Two Jews And Three Opinions

Coming out of a certain cultural milieu, CPE training is usually offered, and experienced in settings where people are "polite:" one does not interrupt someone who is talking, care is taken to not utter critique too hastily, and teachers are always shown due deference. Because of the nature of a traditional Jewish learning context, a CPE group with Jewish students may have a very different "feel" from the usual CPE learning ambience. Because learning in a Jewish context often assumes a spirited "give-and-take" among students and teachers, Jews are more used to asking questions, challenging a teacher/presenter (with due respect), and asserting personal opinions more forcefully.

These are key aspects to the Jewish traditional *hevrutah* (partnership) style of learning. This style of learning assumes that when learners are challenged, everyone's learning and understanding is advanced. Thus, arguments or challenges are not put forth to degrade or humiliate, but rather to get at a deeper meaning and truth. In this context, *not* posing a question may be considered an aloof posture of indifference. Moreover, as a sign of engagement, it is acceptable, even expected, that a listener might interject his/her own ideas or comments,

---

8   As a petitionary prayer, *Shma koleinu* is recited during the morning, afternoon and evening services that occur on weekdays. It is not recited on Shabbat and Holidays.

9   For more on spontaneous prayer and pastoral care, see Gary Lavit's chapter "Promoting Spontaneous Prayer: The Blessings and the Challenges".

as if to say: "I hear you and I want to build on your thinking," or press you to another level of understanding. Yet, even with its benefits, this style can easily be experienced and misunderstood as rude or disrespectful. However, with a group process that is open, this potential "clash of cultural norms" may be yet another opportunity for a rich interfaith exchange.

Supervision

Individual supervision requires creating a relationship of trust and accountability between student and supervisor, as well as a mutual agreement to learn and grow in the experience. While the supervisor of a Jewish CPE program need not be Jewish, he/she does need to have a significant knowledge of Jewish religious practice, culture, and theology in order to help Jewish students achieve their potential. A non-Jewish supervisor needs to be able to expand his/ her own understanding, and hear religious experiences that may be vastly different from what he/she knows. Of course, this also can result in a very rich interfaith dialogue. In addition, it would also be important to amplify the experience of Jewish students inviting other Jewish teachers and chaplains to be guest presenters or additional mentors, to model different styles of Jewish chaplaincy.

Cultural Competence[10]

It is said that the rhythm of Jewish time is what makes Jewish life unique. Each week Jews move from Friday afternoon preparations for Shabbat, then into Shabbat itself, and then back into the week again on Saturday evening. Holidays marking sacred times and historical events punctuate the year. For Jewish CPE students who are observant, this rhythm is integral to their lives, and is often taken for granted when they live immersed in Jewish community. With this in mind, a mixed CPE group that is sensitive to Jewish time can make Jewish participants feel more included.

For nursing home residents as well, the rhythm of the week and the Sabbath may also be important. There can be joy and at times sadness even in times of celebration, i.e. *Shabbat* and the holidays. People experience joy, because of all the rich memories, and the opportunity

---

10   Cf. Susan Buchbinder's chapter "Cultural Competency in a Jewish-sponsored Senior Residential Care Setting".

to sing familiar prayers and evoke timeless customs. People feel sadness at having to leave a beloved home or no longer being an integral part of a community. Certainly, sadness will be felt when close friends and relatives with whom ritual celebrations were shared over the years leave this world. For this reason, the observance of *Yahrzeit* (yearly anniversary of a death), and participating in *Yizkor* (a memorial service for the dead held at certain times of the year) may be very important to residents. Helping residents to reflect, learn, celebrate and mourn during these times can provide tremendous solace. For the resident with dementia, smelling the aroma of traditional holiday cooking, or hearing a certain *nusach* (liturgical melody) for specific holidays can evoke deep and powerful memories.

In addition, those who care for Jewish residents in senior residential care centers would do well to know some modern Jewish history, especially what has occurred over the past century. Without understanding the Holocaust, the formation of the State of Israel, and the exodus of Jews from Russia, a caregiver may not be able to contextualize the experiences related by residents, some of whom may have experienced these events first-hand.[11]

Knowledge of Jewish religious and cultural norms is certainly necessary for providing competent end-of-life care to Jewish residents and their families. It can make all the difference in the world when caregivers as well as the chaplain, are sensitized to the religious and cultural background of a person's life, as well as the family dynamics involved.[12] I recall one resident who in his last weeks started to mourn deeply the death of an infant child early in his life. Apparently, at the time of the child's death, he and his wife had been told that traditional Jewish law did not *require* them to perform the customary mourning rituals for an infant who had not survived beyond thirty days. Consequently, they had never emotionally dealt with this terrible loss, and it had remained with him unresolved. The suggestion of planting a tree in Israel in the name of this infant not only affirmed his lifelong sadness over a life that was felled far too early, but also offered an authentic Jewish way to remember and mark the continuing of the child's memory. This gesture

---

11   On the importance of encouraging staff to know more about modern Jewish history cf. Bev Magidson's chapter "A Connection with Zion: Understanding Jews and Israel".

12   Cf. Jim Jensen's chapter "Being Thy Brother's Keeper: Ministry to People of the Jewish Faith in a Christian Faith-Based Facility".

assisted the resident in finding the peace and closure he needed, while also providing comfort and reassurance to his living children.

Conclusion

At HRC, establishing a Jewish CPE training program has demonstrated how significantly CPE students can contribute to the quality of care provided to patients, staff, and family members. Given our population's overwhelming need for pastoral care grounded in Jewish religious and cultural tenets, we made the conscious choice to create more CPE training opportunities for Jewish chaplaincy students. Our chaplains offer encouragement and support to residents and families as they try to understand, and respond to emotional and spiritual challenges at the end-of-life. They are also present for staff members as they deal with the challenges and losses experienced daily in senior care settings. Looking back on our efforts to create a CPE environment that is truly Jewish in content and process, we are amazed and encouraged by what we have learned, and look forward to sharing it with other CPE training programs.

As HRC works toward realizing its vision of a holistic model of care that includes the physical, emotional and spiritual aspects of health and wellness, chaplaincy will continue to be an essential dimension of the vision. Contributing to its realization, our program hopes to continue to train cadres of rabbis and Jewish professionals who are well-equipped to support and sustain those coping with the travails and tribulations of aging, Jews and non-Jews alike.

Chapter 9

More Battles: Age-Related Challenges For Holocaust Survivors

Paula David, MSW, PhD

Working with aging survivors of the Holocaust and their families is both a challenging and rewarding journey. It is important to learn about the survivor's losses while at the same time never forgetting to celebrate their lives. Working with Holocaust survivors allows us to witness the indefinable potential of the human spirit and its resilient nature. It pushes everyone a little further and a little closer to conceiving the inconceivable and understanding how one can endure the unendurable.

The word "Holocaust" refers to the persecution and mass murder of approximately six million Jews by the Nazi regime between 1938 and 1945. At the end of World War II, over six million Jews had perished. In 1948, The International Refugee Organization was formed to coordinate the care of over 643,000 survivors in displaced persons camps across Europe (USHMM, retrieved 2006). Others managed to leave Europe or found independent shelter with independent agencies or supporters. Today, a Holocaust survivor is defined as any Jew who has lived in a country at the time when it was under Nazi regime, under Nazi occupation, under the regime of Nazi collaborators, as well as any Jew who fled due to the above regime or occupation. As of this writing, this is the definition most commonly in use (AMCHA 2005) and one that recognizes that the emphasis is not on defining a hierarchy of pain and suffering but rather on recognizing an individual's experience of extreme loss and trauma (David, 2002).

With few exceptions, most of those who managed to survive were young adults between the ages of eighteen and thirty-five (Claims

Conference 2005). Those still alive now range in age from their late sixties to their mid-nineties, with some over 100 years of age (David, 2002). Those who managed to survive the trauma and atrocities of the modern world's largest genocide are now facing the last chapter of their own lives. It is unusual to find a cohort that shared such an intense social, historical, moral and personal crisis. Today, they are all older adults dealing with their own aging and mortality.

As issues evolve with their respective mental and physical maturation, so does the need for innovative and resourceful responses. In spite of their shared traumatic Holocaust experience, the aged survivor's mentality and personality today also mirrors the values, behaviors, and expectations of their pre- and post-Holocaust experiences (Davidson, 1992; Rosenbloom, 1985). As survivors age, so does the available research, literature and knowledge. Current literature and practice modalities do not represent the changing needs of those survivors 85 years and older, and their families. Practitioners and policy makers must keep up with these demographic changes in order to provide quality services for these individuals and their families, developing a framework and creative use of theory and practice on a continuum.

The Implications Of The Holocaust Experience For Senior Care

For the first time in the study of genocide survivors in general and Holocaust survivors in particular, we have the opportunity to understand how a cohort of genocide and war survivors have coped with massive trauma across their life course and how it impacts their final years. Holocaust survivors, in order to survive, have had to be cautious of dependency and poor health, often masking or minimizing their needs in order to cope with building new lives after the war. Now, as many face additional challenges of dementia and cognitive loss, it is our mandate to ease the pain as much as possible and ensure the provision of optimum care.

Memory and the ability to remember take on unique elements for survivors. All people are defined by their memories, which provide a frame of reference for worldviews, past, present, and future. It is important to note that while elderly Holocaust survivors must live with their traumatic memories, many also have memories of better times, such as the pre-war years, which may provide solace and reassurance. Both types of memory can leave indelible imprints. The memories of their own children's successes, the pride in grandchildren and the accomplishments of more than sixty post-war years can live alongside the more difficult memories. Positive memories do not erase traumatic and painful ones, but may make living with them easier. Indeed, to lose those memories to dementia is almost an inconceivable loss.

Within the challenges of living with memories of traumatic loss is the potential of losing those memories to age-related dementias. While short- and long-term memory loss would be difficult for anybody, Holocaust survivors coping with cognitive impairment and memory loss may face unique challenges. They can become lost in the very dark labyrinths of older long-term memories of war and trauma. Losing the capacity to sort traumatic memory from positive memory and maintain them in an appropriate or accurate sequential order can make the loss even more painful. As survivors age, more insight into the impact of traumatic memories on cognitively-impaired individuals is developing. When an individual loses his/her ability to differentiate time spans, confuses past and present and conceptualizes the trauma of 60 years ago as happens now, the resulting confusion and pain is felt by all.

Within a senior care setting, one can be alert for triggers that may exacerbate the pain, confusion or sense of time and place of the individual survivor. A trigger is an environmental condition, experience or situation that provokes an adverse physical, emotional or behavioral reaction. For those survivors who are hospitalized or in a long-term care facility, many aspects of the institutional environment may invoke more than one trigger for residents who are survivors.

Triggers can affect survivors, whether or not they have memory impairments. For this reason, all staff members should not only be aware of those that cannot be avoided and their potential negative impact, but also be prepared with a range of responses. Examples of unavoidable triggers that may be present in any health care facility are sounds of somebody crying or screaming, loud voices, sirens, bells, or PA systems. Any one of these could exacerbate very unpleasant memories for the Holocaust survivor, or even cause a more catastrophic reaction.

Awareness of a potential trigger may be more important than its cessation. Awareness and proactive response will allow staff and family to reassure an individual, forewarn an individual where possible, or just be there to keep them as grounded in the present reality as possible.

When one is familiar with environmental triggers, one will also recognize the importance of individualized care. Experience has demonstrated that what may be a trigger for one individual may not be for another. One example of this phenomenon (which had a positive outcome) occurred when a visitor brought a dog as part of a therapeutic pet program to visit a unit for cognitively-impaired residents. An alert staff member, remembering that many survivors were traumatized by Nazi guard and attack dogs, saw the dog as a potential trigger and immediately went to stay with a particular survivor so she wouldn't notice the dog. The woman was severely impaired and had been nonverbal for months. She heard the commotion surrounding the dog's visit, and before the staff member could reach her room, the woman saw the group and the dog at the end of the hall and actually ran towards them. She got down on her knees, embraced the animal and started speaking to the dog in Hungarian. After talking with the family, staff learned that, as a child, the woman had owned a puppy of the same breed. The dog became a weekly visitor to the unit and to this particular woman for the rest of her life. Indeed, the dog was a trigger, but a very positive one for this woman, as it brought back a whole flood of fond memories. The lesson here is the importance of not making assumptions about what might or might not be a trigger for a particular individual.

Showers are another trigger that may initiate traumatic memories for many survivors. During the Holocaust, a survivor, currently living in a senior care facility, may have witnessed his/her entire family march into "showers" and then gassed to death. Thus, it would be fair to assume that this person may have a strong reaction to a present-day institutional shower. On the other hand, the reality may be that this person enjoys and looks forward to his shower, appreciating how it leaves him refreshed and clean. Other survivors, who may never have been in a concentration camp, may still identify so strongly with the connection between gas chambers and showers, that the thought of a shower or having a second person take them to a shower is a strong trigger. The potential connection, flash-back or associative memory can precipitate anything from emotional discomfort to a catastrophic reaction. All caregivers need to be aware of the more common triggers (http://www.baycrest.org/HolocaustSurvivors/triggers.pdf), and appreciate that they may conjure up uniquely individual memories among survivors. It is also important to remember that triggers may cause reactions that are expected as well as those that are unexpected, and that anything may cause an individual to relive his/her traumatic experiences. The challenge lies in being prepared for the reaction that is unexpected, and to support those vulnerable older adults who have lived through extreme trauma in their early years.

Because there are few if any reference points for understanding the full range and extent of suffering experienced by victims of the Holocaust, the emotional responses of social workers or other professionals to such massive devastation is an ever-present factor in counseling survivors and their descendants. Many survivors endured levels of physical, emotional and sexual abuse well beyond the scope of any preparatory academic training. Regardless of their individual wartime experiences, Holocaust survivors share the experience of assaults on personal freedom, dignity and identity. Based on work with aging survivors, a better understanding of the emotional impact of extreme trauma on the client, the family and the professionals who care for them is emerging.

A difficult notion for modern health care providers to assimilate is that there are many conditions that we cannot heal or correct. Experience with aging survivors demonstrates that there is no perspective, process or amount of time that will erase the trauma of genocide. That older survivors may actually feel their losses more intensely as they age is also becoming more apparent. Therefore, as we work with this diminishing cohort, our emphasis should be on what we can provide for them, and how we can ensure that they live their final years with as little trauma and as much dignity as possible. As we strive to maintain dignity for those in a life stage that can be undignified, in healthcare systems that often forget the importance of dignity to human well-being, this is a challenge in itself.

Living With Loss

The study of aging encompasses the study of death and dying, bereavement and loss. Death concludes the last chapter of a person's life and chaplains working in senior care facilities are called upon to support residents and families during this critical time. For the current cohort of older adults who grew up in an era of shorter life expectancies and fewer medical interventions, this is a very different experience from what they might have anticipated. For Holocaust survivors who equate death with traumatic loss, what they anticipate may be even more foreign and therefore more frightening. For many of their children, this may be their first experience dealing with the loss of an older relative and they may experience similar difficulties.

Families of Holocaust survivors often have fewer resources and less experience with issues of death and dying. It is a strange irony that this group of adult children, intimately knowledgeable about the death of so many, often experiences the death of an elderly parent as shrouded in mystery. Thus, mental health professionals and caregivers must be cognizant of the unique sensitivities and vulnerabilities of this group when discussing prognoses, end-of-life directives and bereavement issues in general.

Pastoral care can be helpful by offering elements of psychosocial education, counseling, advocacy and support in navigating the appropriate health care system. As discussions about survivors' end-of-life issues emerge, there are specific moral, spiritual and social issues that individuals or families might want to discuss with chaplains and other pastoral caregivers, as well as systemic, logistical and legal information that they may require. Like other mental health professionals, those involved in providing pastoral care for survivors and their families must also be aware of the impact of early life trauma on later life, as well as relevant cultural issues and family dynamics in order to provide sensitive and appropriate support.

Within Judaism, there is a comprehensive set of rituals, customs and traditional observances to support individuals and families through the bereavement process (Berlat and Strauss, 2006). Time has demonstrated to generations of Jewish families that the traditions of immediate burial, specific mourning prayers and burial rituals followed by sitting *shiva* (the observance of seven days of mourning for immediate family members) provides solace to the bereaved family and friends. These observances are meant to honor the memory of the dead and to support the mourners through the period immediately following the death, so that they can make the transition from loss to life, from sorrow and alienation to once again being part of the community. While religious affiliation within Judaism may generate some alternate interpretations of the various customs, they are remarkably similar and consistent throughout the Jewish community.

From the first anticipation of death, to the preparation and care of the body, to burial, mourning and memorializing of the deceased, Jewish traditions and customs associated with death and dying create a structure and a sense of normalization in the face of upset and disruption. However, for many Holocaust survivors these rituals do not begin to provide the comfort and solace historically associated with them – comfort and solace which non-survivors might take for granted. For example, reciting the Mourner's *Kaddish*, the Jewish prayer for honoring the dead which focuses on praising God (yet has no references to death and dying) may prove exceptionally challenging for the survivor who questions the role or presence of God in the Holocaust. The strength of the *shiva* experience comes from mourners being surrounded by family and friends who attend to them through their grieving. Yet, many survivor families have small circles of friends and even smaller family circles. For these families, the circle may prove inadequate in its capacity to provide comfort, and mourning the loss of one may trigger mourning the loss of many.

Jewish practice also involves regular visits to the cemetery where traditional prayers and memorials are recited at various times throughout the calendar year, on the anniversary of the death, and on designated Jewish holidays. Within survivor families, loved ones' dates of death are often unknown as are, in many cases, the actual circumstances of death. Furthermore, the location of the remains of family members lost in the Holocaust is a painful consideration: at best these locations are unknown, and at worst it is known or assumed that the remains are in one or more of the mass burial sites across Europe, or in the mountainous piles of ashes on the sites of the former death camps. Jewish cemeteries in the post World War II world do not symbolize eternal rest for Holocaust survivors.

Still, survivors often hold on to traditions that once resonated with them. To be sure, this can also present challenges to a "normal" mourning process. An Ashkenazi[1] Jewish custom is to name a new baby after a dead relative to honor that person's memory and ensure that it remains alive as part of the family legacy. Often children of survivors carry several names of murdered relatives, so that the honor of memory also becomes a *burden* of memory.

Because Jewish customs and traditions that traditionally support mourners are often woefully inadequate for Holocaust survivors, many families are creating new and innovative ways to cope with Holocaust-related multiple deaths and their painful memories as well as current spousal and parental deaths. In the course of my work with survivors and their families, I have seen the results of these efforts. Many Jewish cemeteries have memorial stones with the deceased survivor's epitaph

---

1   "Ashkenazi" refers to the Jewish communities of Western, Central and Eastern Europe. "*Ashkenaz*" is the biblical Hebrew word for the area now encompassing Germany and France.

on one side, and on the reverse a list of immediate family members who perished in the Holocaust. In this way, the post-war family has a permanent marker and a place to perform the traditional mourning rites for those relatives murdered by the Nazis. In addition, some cemeteries have erected sculptures, stones or other decorative pieces to list family names, town names or pay tribute to the memories and loss of whole groups of murdered people. Holocaust survivors and their families continue to grapple with how to adapt typical traditional rituals and customs in order to accommodate their atypical mourning needs.

Synagogues are also recognizing this need and many have incorporated special prayers for the murdered six million Jews within the framework of traditional holy day and memorial services. Jewish communities all over the world are still coming to terms with this catastrophe, and developing new forms of memorializing the victims of the Holocaust (Danieli 1994, David 2007), even while the survivors are contemplating their own mortality. Modern Jewry's paradoxical familiarity with the death of millions juxtaposed with their lack of exposure to normal aging and death – combined with their collective identity as "survivors" in a post-Auschwitz age – has contributed to a different view of mortality and loss.

Seeking Understanding From Those Who Weren't There

Rosenbloom (1983) identifies larger issues connected to the Holocaust and wrote her seminal article intending "to stimulate engagement with the moral and universal issues of the Holocaust," and recognize how the survivors "unique historic experience has rarely been given attention" (p.205). She speaks to the importance of "the political and moral lessons to be derived from study of the Holocaust," and writes, "(I)ncreasingly, there is recognition that these lessons are crucial, perhaps vital, to our survival as a people and as a civilization" (p.206).

This need to understand exists on both macro and micro levels. The political and moral lessons for social workers noted by Rosenbloom (1983) are further underlined by the tragic reality of recurring wars and genocides. The post-Holocaust genocides in Cambodia, Yugoslavia, the Balkans, Rwanda and Darfur have generated new interest in the life course of survivors of Europe's Holocaust from the media and helping professions. Rosenbloom (1994), in her discussion of what we can learn from the Holocaust, states: "The lessons of the Holocaust are vital and universal, timely and timeless" (p.1).

While every trauma survivor's story is unique, the common theme is one of loss and pain. The differences range through countries of origin, language, pre-war lives, war experiences and post-war coping skills. Chaplains and other care providers would do well to be prepared to accommodate survivors' unique vulnerabilities as they cope with age-related losses and illnesses, and respond with programs, policies and care interventions that are sensitive to their needs. Indeed, there is no retroactive justice for this particular group, but there is a moral need for an agency- and community-wide responsiveness that is systemic, immediate and sensitive. While the wrongs of the past cannot be reversed, there is still time and opportunity for senior care providers to ensure that aging Holocaust survivors can end their lives with the kind of compassionate care that honors their unique experiences and their common dignity.

References

AMCHA. (2005). "National Israeli Center for Psychosocial Support of Survivors of the Holocaust and the Second Generation." Retrieved March 2005, from http://amcha.org

Berlat, N. and A. J. Strauss (2006). "Engaging eternity: A Jewish approach to death, dying, grief and bereavement" *International Journal of Health Promotion and Education* 44(1).

Claims Conference. (2005). "Jewish Material War Claims Against Germany Inc." Retrieved June 2005, from http://claimscon.org.

Danieli, Y. (1994). " As Survivors Age: An Overview, Part I and II." *Clinical Quarterly* 4 (1 & 2).

David, P., Ed., (2008) "Caring for Aging Holocaust Survivors, A Practice Manual", Baycrest, Retrieved July 2008, from www.baycrest.org/holocaustsurvivors

David, P. (2002). "Aging Survivors of the Holocaust: Unique Needs, Responses and Long-Term Group Work Approaches." *Journal of Social Work in Long-term Care,* 1(3), New York, Haworth.

David, P. (2007). Issues of Death and Dying for Adult Children of Holocaust Survivors, in *Dying and Death.* A. Kasher Ed., Rodopi Press.

Davidson, S. (1992). *Holding on to Humanity: The Message of Holocaust Survivors: the Shamai Davidson Papers.* New York.

Rosenbloom, M. (1983). "Implications of the Holocaust for Social Work." *Social Casework: The Journal of Contemporary Social Work.*: 205-213.

Rosenbloom, M. (1994). What Can We Learn from the Holocaust?, *Occasional Papers in Jewish History and Thought.* H. College. New York,

Hunter College Jewish Social Studies Program.

Rosenbloom, M. (1985). "The Holocaust Survivor in Late Life." *Gerontological Social Work Practice in the Community*: 181-190.

USHMM, United States Holocaust Memorial Museum, (2006) Holocaust Encyclopedia, United Nations Relief and Rehabilitation Association, retrieved July 2006, http://www.ushmm.org/wlc/en/

Chapter 10
Jewish Chaplaincy In The Green House Model Of Care

Rabbi Karen Landy, Rabbi Sara Paasche-Orlow

Hebrew Rehabilitation Center in Dedham, MA, is a 250-bed chronic care hospital for senior care opened in the fall of 2009. Its approach to senior residential care is based on the Green House model. In this chapter we will examine the unique role of the chaplain in this particular model of care as it is developing at this new facility. Of the seniors we serve in long-term care, 80% use Medicaid and 85% of our population is Jewish. Most residents are English speaking, with some knowledge of Yiddish, and are from Boston and the surrounding area.

The Green House model of care was developed by Dr. William Thomas in 2002. It is premised on the idea that senior care environments should not be based on a medical model but rather on the creation of a home-like environment. In the traditional medical model of care, facilities are designed to accommodate staff functions. For example, the central organizing principle of the medical ward is to manage medication administration and other nursing services. The nurses' station serves as the central hub and almost all parameters of the daily experience are circumscribed by the medication and meal deliveries. The Green House model, in contrast, aspires to shift the architectural and cultural focus of the living space from staff functions to a resident-oriented environment. Residents live in "Households" with an open kitchen, living room, and dining room in the center. Around this central living area, there are rooms for fourteen to sixteen residents. The daily schedule is flexible, with residents waking and eating according to individual routines.

In the Green House model, meals are planned and served in

the Households. In our version, staff members cook breakfast in the Households according to the residents' wishes. For lunch and dinner warming trays with food are brought to the Households, and the community eats together family style. Family members can bring and prepare food with the residents and can easily join in meals. Two of the 15 Households are kosher, so residents have the option to live in a kosher community.[1]

The staff is trained to work in teams with shared responsibilities and with the care of the resident at the center of these responsibilities. In contrast to the traditional medical model of care, the role of the resident assistant (RA) is central in the day-to-day life of the resident and therefore empowered to help foster each resident's autonomy and independence. Similarly, the chaplain is part of each Household team.

The goal here is to create an environment that feels more like a home and not a medical institution. In this environment, no medical equipment or charts are visible and emergency medical systems are discretely positioned behind sliding paintings in resident rooms. In sync with efforts being made throughout senior care, there is an emphasis on the elimination of unnecessary medications and schedule simplification. In addition, staff tries to ensure that health care appointments and therapies do not get in the way of individuals' activities and other commitments.

Household staff are expected to get to know each resident, his/her care plan, wellness goals, and to familiarize themselves with each resident's interests and hobbies. In addition to larger group programs in music and art, there are small group activities on each Household based on the interests of the Household members.

According to the late Jewish theologian Mordecai Kaplan, there are three components of Jewish identity: belonging, behavior, and belief.[2]

---

1   Editors' note: Cf. notes 14 and 16 in Cary Kozberg's chapter "You Shall Be Holy: The Roles of the Jewish Chaplain in Senior Residential Care Settings". As Nathaniel Popper notes in his article "Bowing to Market, Consumer Demand, Some Jewish Nursing Homes Go Treyf" (*Forward,* January 27, 2010), observance of *kashrut* (Jewish dietary laws) is not the *a sine qua non* it used to be in most senior residential care facilities under Jewish auspices. At HRC, abiding by the rules of *kashrut* is an option for residents rather than a mandatory policy.

2   Neil Gillman, *Sacred Fragments* (Philadelphia: The Jewish Publication Society, 1990), xvii.

Kaplan understood *belonging* to a people as the dominant feature of Jewish identity. He defined *behavior* as the choices that people make about how they live their lives. In transitioning from one's home to a new residence in a senior care facility, people can regain a sense of "rootedness" by talking about their lives to new staff and new neighbors – talking about choices made and significant people. Once an individual feels more rooted, he/she can find ways to become an active member of the new community, and in the process affirm old *beliefs* – or assimilate new ones – which imbue this new life with meaning.

We will use Kaplan's model as the organizing principle for this chapter, for it describes the model of pastoral care which has been developed at HRC's Green Houses. In Section One, we look at the first stages of a resident's transition to living in a Household. A new resident's involvement with the chaplain often focuses on finding a sense of belonging in the new environment. Section Two will discuss the role of the chaplain in helping residents to experience a new life phase. The chaplain works with residents on life review and learns about each individual resident, and how that person's life has had meaning up to this point. The chaplain serves as a transitional bridge to this new existence. Sections Three, Four and Five concentrate on how the chaplain responds to a resident's "beliefs" and personal values. The chaplain helps fosters ways of finding meaning as people address end-of-life concerns, create new relationships, and manage the challenges of illness and the waning of life.

Transitioning Into A Small Community: The Chaplain As Community And Culture Builder

When residents begin to live together as a Household "group", a culture begins to emerge. Living together and eating around a large table for lunch and dinner, people get to know each other, make friends, and cultivate areas of common interest and discourse (i.e., sports, current events, politics, and movies). Staff facilitates conversations at meal times. Based on the individuals and their experiences as a group, each Household creates rituals that in turn result in the creation of a unique community. For example, one Household bakes birthday cakes and celebrates every resident and staff birthday. Each cake is made according to the tastes and preferences of the individual. This is a way for residents and staff to create a sense of commonality and connectedness with one another.

The chaplain is one of the guides for creating the cultural norms of a Household. For example, when the men on one Household expressed the desire to eat their meals separately from the women, the chaplain helped arrange for two separate eating groups. The men felt more natural and at ease in the company of other men, and were able to discuss more freely their interests when they had their own space.

The chaplain also helps staff integrate new residents by translating and explaining cultural norms that may be unfamiliar. She supports staff by encouraging RAs to take time to get to know a newcomer, and at times facilitates this by prompting the RA and then filling in as needed so that he/she can spend time sitting and talking with the resident and thus build a relationship.

Meanwhile, the chaplain moves throughout the building and spends time with residents who may have experienced a critical event over the past 24 hours, offering support to family and care staff. Emergent care needs can interfere with and disturb the equilibrium of a community. The chaplain assists in helping Households handle these spontaneous upheavals as she counsels people, and support families that are present. In this way, she assists in keeping these situations from escalating and thus putting more stress on the Household communities:

From the Chaplain's notes:[3] The day Mrs. L moved in, she was anxious about her new home. She had lived on her own for the past 20 years, but after she had a fall, her family realized she needed more help. She had become very isolated and needed more social interactions. I came to see her during her first meal with her Household. Everyone around the table introduced themselves and enjoyed sharing their experiences. Often this sharing leads to the discovery of shared connections and experiences, as it quickly becomes apparent that many of the residents' lives have overlapped in certain places, at certain times. Mrs. L. discovered that some residents were from her former neighborhood and were familiar with her community, and that they even had some friends in common.

When the meal was over, I asked Mrs. L if she wanted me to put a mezuzah on her door. She gladly accepted my offer. I invited her two neighbors to join us. We all gathered by her room, recited the blessings and put the mezuzah up. Then I asked the others if they wanted to offer Mrs. L their own

---

3   This and all subsequent passages in italics are "Chaplain's Notes," written by Rabbi Karen Landy.

blessings. I smiled as they said "health" and "a new home."[4]

These initial interactions make people feel at home in a new place, and welcomed by a community that will soon become for them a very special subset of peers. The ritual of hanging a mezuzah, creating a home for an individual, and doing this in a supportive community, helped Mrs. L begin to better acclimate and feel at home.

"I am not going home": The Chaplain As Transitional Bridge

Often, after the initial experience of moving into a Household, when family members have begun to return to their own lives, new residents may experience feelings of sadness and loss as they fully realize what they have left behind. This is frequently augmented by the death of beloved friends and family. As is the case with most moves to senior residential care facilities, people have left homes containing a lifetime of belongings, where they have lived for many years. In addition, the move itself may have been caused by a decline in their health. In responding to such circumstances, the chaplain can listen, acknowledge the loss and bear witness to a person's pain. Initial conversations with residents always reveal a personal narrative. Some of a resident's story may be shared with the chaplain in the presence of a family member, especially when the resident is not fully verbal, or is experiencing dementia or delirium. Through this narrative, a fuller story and personality of the individual begins to emerge for the chaplain. Certainly it can be a meaningful moment not only for the chaplain, but also for residents and their families: in hearing their own words, the resident's personal identity is affirmed and enhanced.

Learning a new resident's life story, the chaplain can share the person's interests with other staff, so that what is learned about the person is integrated into the larger culture of the Household, thus helping the culture itself to evolve. It is essential that at least one member of the team get to know each newcomer in depth. Getting to know newcomers includes becoming aware of people who have been close to them, what they have done in the course of their lives, and what events have shaped their lives. Again, this knowledge is used to

---

4   While there is a mezuzah on the external door of the building, HRC affirms the right of each resident to choose whether or not to put a mezuzah on the door to his/her own room.

weave what is important to them into the fabric of the new life they are beginning. A resident's personal pictures and objects can be extremely helpful in helping the community itself choose books, games, music, and art for the common areas:

Within a few days of each new resident's arrival, I make a visit to his/ her room. This initial visit often includes the resident giving me a "a tour of the pictures" and sharing the stories attached to each photograph. Listening attentively and asking questions is one of the ways that I as chaplain, experience the privilege, honor, and responsibility of getting to know each resident.

When Mrs. L moved in, I went to her room to welcome her, and asked her to tell me a bit about her life. I asked her to tell me about the photographs that surrounded her as well as those few precious pieces of furniture and tchatchkes (sentimental objects) that she and her family had chosen to bring along. As she spoke, it became apparent that each piece had been selected for its special story. Old pictures of grandparents from Poland, a favorite vase that had been given to her by her husband 60 years ago, a letter from her five-year-old great grandson – each was a touchstone that helped her feel at home.

Visiting residents' rooms and learning the importance of each object that they have chosen to bring is like making a journey into their souls. For some people the move to a senior care facility may be one of many; for others it may be a move from the home in which they lived for over fifty years and where they raised their families. As the chaplain hears these individual stories, her experience of the individual becomes deeper and fuller. These stories can be a powerful aid for the chaplain to affirm the resident's uniqueness back to him/her, as well as in the larger resident community.

Some Households have created rituals that help residents get to know one another better and to build stronger communal ties among them. For one Household, Wednesday afternoon is when each resident is asked to bring to the dining room table something from their room. At some point, during refreshments, each resident has the opportunity to talk about the object he/she brought. As the stories behind the objects are shared, the residents quickly become aware of some significant connections which they share. Indeed, some of these moments seem like "mini-reunions": when one resident brought out a picture of her high school class, another resident realized that both of them had graduated from the same school and had mutual friends.

On the other hand, sometimes the sharing creates connections based on shared sorrow. Many residents have lived through numerous losses. Some have not only outlived their immediate family and friends, but may have also buried children and grandchildren. For some, such gatherings may be their opportunity to share these stories. It is often in these smaller circles, around the dining room table, that residents will articulate these losses and reach out to others around the table. Experiencing loss and bereavement is a part of aging, and a special feature of living in a community of elders is having others around who have had similar experiences. By creating pathways of support among individuals and eliciting responses that offer comfort, recall blessings, and foster resilience, the chaplain can shepherd the group through these moments of sadness, and ensure that no one feels isolated.

"I've lived my life, I'm ready to die": The Chaplain As Witness And Advocate

No human being goes through life without experiencing loss and thus every human being must face what loss brings in its wake. The role of the chaplain is to be present for the individual who is experiencing the sadness brought about by significant loss, support his/her strategies for staying resilient (which may encourage the inclusion of certain spiritual practices) and ensure that however a resident responds to loss, he/she will not experience it alone. As people age and become more frail some may experience a deep sense of personal isolation. Living in a communal setting provides opportunities to make new friends, and re-engage in the activities that were once meaningful. Music, art, literature, current events, prayer services, and Torah study can all help a person find renewed meaning and serve as a vehicle for feeling more connected to a purposeful life again:

At 97 years old, Mrs. L had outlived all her siblings and her friends. Last week, her son revealed that he had cancer and that he would be having treatment. The son approached me, the chaplain because he wanted to make sure his mom got some extra care. When I came to visit Mrs. L she looked at me and cried. After a few minutes she asked "Why?" and then proceeded to talk about her life and how she had lived a full life and now was tired. Chaplains are called on to be vessels for holding both a person's sadness and joy, acknowledging that both are present and necessary in life. Mrs. L wanted to support her son by being strong and by praying for strength and healing. So we prayed.

Indeed, even in the most trying times, people can show the most amazing resilience. There are many examples of people like Mrs. L who, after a tragic loss, continue to express their sadness, mark it regularly with rituals, cherish the memories, and still find ways to live their lives with purpose by helping other people, making new friends, and engaging in meaningful activities.

Unfortunately, there are others who, when facing difficult health outcomes and physical suffering, decide that their life is over; they have reached the conclusion that there is nothing left to live for or look forward to, and that they are ready to leave this world. As part of a Household team, the chaplain may be the most appropriate team member to work with residents and families to make sure that the resident's end-of-life directives are clear and that they reflect his/her beliefs and values. Ideally, the family should be comfortable with the resident's decisions. When this is not the case, the chaplain can play a unique role in working toward reconciliation when there are differing beliefs and desires. Often, having one's wishes about end-of-life issues accepted by one's family and caregivers helps a person to live the final days without anxiety and fear of disempowerment and thus perhaps embrace life a little longer. In other situations, especially when there is a quick deterioration and decline, a person may be cared for simply by being accompanied in their dying. To be sure, this can be very hard on the members and staff of the person's Household. When death becomes more imminent for a member of the household, it is the choice of other residents whether or not to be a part of their neighbor's dying process. In such moments, the chaplain can play a significant facilitating role in helping the group to respond by giving and receiving blessings and to say good-bye.

Forming Friendships, Creating Shared Moments: The Chaplain as Matchmaker

As people in the Households get to know each other and form relationships among themselves, connections emerge that strengthen over time. One role that may be important for the chaplain to play is that of "people connector" – bringing folks together who can benefit from each other's friendship, and share a sense of common purpose:

One of Mrs. L's most precious possessions was her Scrabble set. I noticed this immediately upon her arrival. When I asked her about it, she told me that she and her husband had played weekly with another couple, a routine that had lasted for three decades. She proudly showed me her very-used paperback dictionary which went hand in hand with the game board. I mentioned to Mrs. L that there was a Scrabble group (organized by a volunteer) meeting every Wednesday morning. She smiled and said, "I haven't played in a while but I think I remember." After a few weeks of the group meeting on Wednesdays, they realized that they could organize a game during the weekend. The group decided to meet on Saturday afternoons. Since the members of the group all attended Shabbat morning services, the chaplain included in the announcements at the end of the service the formation of the new Shabbat afternoon Scrabble club. Similar arrangements were made for the bridge and poker clubs. Residents are eager to connect with one another and to discover new friends who have common interests.

Jewish and American holidays are celebrated on each Household, with families joining in the observances, and special foods being cooked together in the communal kitchens. Shabbat services and meals are also times for Households to come together and find a special joy and sense of peace associated with Shabbat. There are multiple ways of celebrating: as families gather, together with a Household, or at times by themselves. These celebrations are affirmations of time-honored customs and beliefs that shape, and are at the core of people's identities:

Passover is a time for families to gather together to share the story of the Exodus from Egyptian slavery over a ritual Seder meal served with traditional symbolic foods. Indeed Passover is a holiday when it is important to have a "family" atmosphere. In order to respond appropriately, each Household prepared for the holiday with a discussion on family traditions and recipes. It is important that the staff participate in such discussions and hear what residents have to say, not necessarily with the goal of replicating traditions but merely to appreciate them and honor the feelings with which they are discussed. As the holiday approached, residents eagerly noticed the traditional Passover foods coming up from the kitchen. Together with the staff, they began to put the traditional food items on the Passover Seder plate and set the Passover table. When it came to participating in the Seders, there were many options: Some family members joined in to lead Seders with the Household communities. Other residents chose to have their own family

Seder in a private room at the Center, or to join in a large communal Seder. Many of the residents' memories of the holiday were captured and brought to life in the atmosphere created in each Household.

In The Valley Of The Shadow: The Chaplain As Shepherd

One of the most challenging aspects of the chaplain's job is to help residents and staff in each Household deal with a resident's imminent death. A chaplain's facilitation of conversation can prepare the group for the expected loss, and help the community in saying good-bye. During such moments, the chaplain works to keep the emotional equilibrium of the environment as stable as possible, checking in with staff and providing emotional space and permission for staff to share their feelings. In senior residential care communities, families often become attached to each other and to the residents, and these connections are only enhanced when there is good communication and support, particularly in times of stress and high anxiety. When a resident does pass away, emails are sent to all the families of that resident's Household with funeral information so that they may pay their respects.

In the Green House model of care, residents and families have a greater degree of independence and control over their care choices, in contrast to the traditional types of care often associated with traditional long-term care institutions. One example of this greater degree of control is that residents whose health conditions change are not automatically sent to the hospital. Instead of being sent to the emergency room or being admitted directly into the hospital, the vast majority of our residents choose to be treated by the nurses and doctors available to the Household. Thus, when a person's condition worsens, the interdisciplinary team, consisting of medical staff, the social worker, and the chaplain all focus on the resident and his/her family. What is offered is an approach to care (and healing!) that is more holistic than what would be offered in a typical hospital setting. Moreover, if the chaplain knows the resident and has created a relationship of trust and mutual respect with the resident, the time of "saying good-bye" can be one of blessing and a peaceful letting-go for all involved:

Mr. W was 94 years old. All his life he had been a community builder. From the moment he moved into our facility he wanted to make a difference. He was always smiling and introducing himself to everyone. Within a short time of his arrival, he decided to begin two projects on his own: the first was to collect everyone's birthdays and the second was to form a committee that would organize celebrations of these days. He found a few other volunteers who were willing to hand deliver birthday cards and also sing birthday greetings. But more than anything, Mr. W wanted to create a residents' newsletter. With the help of staff, he organized a committee which now puts out a monthly newspaper featuring a list of birthdays, upcoming events, "getting to know you" articles, interviews and highlights of past events. To be sure, while such an undertaking might be common in an independent living community, the level of independence and autonomy it reflects in a skilled nursing environment may be a bit unusual.

Gradually, Mr. W's health began to decline. He was diagnosed with terminal cancer and eventually it became clear to all that he had only a few weeks to live. Both the doctor and chaplain were present to share this news with Mr. W's family and then with him. After the doctor left, the chaplain sat with Mr. W and they began to talk about what was in store. It was clear that before he passed from this world, he wanted to share and celebrate his life. Within a day, the newspaper committee organized a gathering for Mr. W where he was presented with the title "Editor-in-Chief" and given a framed copy of the first edition of the newspaper. Mr. W made the group promise that they would continue to do good work.

Mr. W spent the next few days with his family and friends. In addition, staff often came for final visits to his room. As chaplain, I was called on to support other residents and staff as they faced his impending passing, and spent time sitting with Mr. W reading to him, singing with him, and supporting his family.

The true effectiveness of this model of care lies in its creating and nurturing of an intimate relationship among residents, staff and family members. Families become very attached to other residents and other families. When a resident dies, the sense of loss is multi-faceted and felt in many ways by many people. Shortly after Mr. W's funeral, his family returned to the Center so that we could celebrate his life, and share memories and our gratitude for having known him.

Conclusion

The vision of care associated with the Green House model strives to sustain residents' independence and vitality. As a result, the role of the geriatric care chaplain is expanded to enable the interdisciplinary health care team to attend to all parts of a person's life. When this happens, the model stays true to Mordecai Kaplan's three components of Jewish identity: belonging, behavior, belief. Residents are helped and encouraged to express the values and events that have shaped their personal identities so that each individual can experience a full sense of belonging to, and being known in the community. This vision of care facilitates relationships among all involved in the life of the Household – residents, family members and staff – so that residents' activities and daily life choices are consistent with the activities and choices that were a part of their lives before they became residents. Affirming such choices also includes helping residents articulate their healthcare wishes and making sure that these choices accurately reflect their personal and deeply-held beliefs and are therefore respected. And finally, this vision of care is about creating meaningful norms and practices for the Household community itself – norms and practices that will be rooted in, and enthusiastically promote resilience and hope for all who are a part of it.

Part Two ~ Pastoral Programming

Chapter 11

Grief And Mourning In Senior Residential Care: A Jewish Pastoral Framework

Sheila Segal, BCC

I was taken by surprise when Bertha asked if it would be possible to have her funeral in the synagogue of our long-term care center. It was during an Oneg Shabbat (Sabbath fellowship hour) *following Saturday morning services, and a small group of residents had been talking about the* aufruf *(pre-nuptial calling to the Torah) of Rhoda's grandson celebrated that morning. The happy occasion reminded them of other recent family* simchas *(celebrations) held at the Center – the naming ceremony for Yetta's great-granddaughter, the* sheva brachot *(seven blessings of marriage) for Izzy's youngest son. The residents were saying how wonderful it is when they can share each other's* nachas *(joy) and participate in all kinds of life cycle events.*

"You know, I was wondering if we could have a funeral here as well," Bertha suddenly interjected. "I've lived here for three years," she explained, "and this is my community." She said it would be comforting to her to know that her friends and caregivers would be able to attend. The other residents agreed that it would be a good thing. Like most of us, they would not want to miss the opportunity to attend a friend's funeral. But what, they wondered, did the chaplain think?[1]

Bertha's request was startling and challenging. While we may agree that it's important for elders to participate in all kinds of life cycle events, and that we should extend ourselves to host such events in nursing home settings, the prospect of having funerals on site pushes the comfort zone of many Jewish senior care facilities. The responses are predictable: "*We don't want people to think that this is*

---

1   Vignettes in italics are actual situations that I encountered when I worked as a chaplain, though names have been changed to respect confidentiality.

a place where you come to die." "It would be too upsetting for our residents and families." "We're not a funeral home." Very few would actually permit a funeral with the casket present to take place. Some are reluctant even to have memorial services or to post a death notice.

Nursing homes and other senior residential facilities do not want to be thought of as places where people come to die, and many people find it hard to deal with the fact of living or working in a place where death occurs frequently. But the reality is impossible to deny. As people live longer, the resident population of senior care facilities becomes older and frailer, and hospital stays become shorter, death is an even more frequent and pervasive presence in the daily lives of residents and their caregivers. The truth is that, with the exception of those who come for short-term rehabilitation, most elders who come to live in a nursing home will die in a nursing home. While many still prefer to treat these deaths as hushed events, the obligation to meet the spiritual needs of residents, as well as those of their families and caregivers, requires those of us who work in senior residential care to acknowledge this truth and help those touched by these deaths to prepare for what they will bring in their wake.

The answer to Bertha's question depends in large measure on whether we have the courage to do so. Her request is a poignant statement of three important spiritual needs of elders: the need to feel physically and spiritually connected to a community; the need to mourn their losses; and the need to anticipate, even plan for, their own death. Meeting these needs is a challenge to all work in the field of senior residential care, and especially to chaplains.

Something Sacred Happens Here

"There is a time to be born and a time to die." The well-known words of Ecclesiastes (3:2) remind us that living and dying are really not separate events but interwoven experiences. There is no place on earth where death is not an integral part of the life of the community, and from the wisdom of the Jewish tradition we know that how we respond to death, as individuals and as a community, has a major impact on the way we continue to live our lives. This is as true for a community of elders as it is for any other Jewish community.

Senior care chaplains who are well-versed in the Jewish approach to death and mourning can help create a community in which losses are openly acknowledged, so that grief may be expressed and shared by residents, family members, and caregivers. For those who fear that being open about death is too upsetting to residents, it is important to remember that avoidance is disrespectful of both the deceased and their survivors. The absence of public acknowledgement of such losses can also result in the emotional complications of "disenfranchised grief," grief that is neither validated nor expressed. This is a syndrome that can afflict many caregivers and residents, causing them to pull back from relationships, lose interest in activities, or become easily irritated.

Martha, a nurse in a dementia special care unit, was feeling enormous stress and sadness after a month when several of her residents died. Martha was so enervated that she decided to take a 10-day break, essentially to give herself space to grieve. When another death occurred shortly after her return, the chaplain came to offer her personal condolences. Martha's appreciation was effusive: "Thank you so much for noticing that it hurts. It really helps to hear someone say that."

It is natural – and basic – for Jewish chaplains to validate the pain of loss. More importantly, we help our co-workers find meaning in the pain if we foster a climate in which death is regarded as a sacred passage and care of the dying is valued as sacred work. Beginning with orientation of new staff, we need to speak about the emotional challenges of working in a place where death happens so frequently and emphasize that what they as caregivers do during the last weeks or hours of a resident's life can really make a substantive difference in how the death occurs and how family and loved ones respond.

Letting go can be difficult for caregivers. One way of easing this difficulty may be to share the Jewish view that there comes a time when it is not our human role to intervene in the dying process but our responsibility, and our privilege, to promote comfort. As residents approach the end of life, we can remind frontline caregivers of their important role in creating an atmosphere that nurtures trust, peace, and the expression of love that is rooted in their intimate knowledge of, and attachment to, these individuals.

As spiritual caregivers, we ourselves enhance the sanctity of this passage through the quality of presence and listening that we provide as well as through our offerings of psalms, prayers, and religious melodies. We show others how to create a peaceful, sacred space by doing little things such as turning off the TV, opening the shades to natural light, introducing some relaxing music, and refraining from needless "chatter" to allow moments of silence. At the same time, we can remind others that the dying person may still be able to hear until the very end, that their own words or songs will provide comfort, and that there is still time to say whatever needs to be said.

In addition, it is important to explain to caregivers that at the time of death a window is opened to mark the beginning of the soul's return to God, a candle (albeit electric) is lit as a sign of God's watchful presence, and a simple white sheet drawn over the deceased as a sign of holiness and respect. Sitting at the bedside, reading psalms or talking quietly with family and caregivers, we resist the tendency to "spring into action", taking time to simply honor the mystery of this life transition and the privilege granted to all who have participated and witnessed it.

The Need To Know

Milton, Dorothy, and Freda were wondering what happened to their friend Ann, who lived in the same "household" of their nursing home. They had not seen her for several days. Because of her congestive heart failure, Ann had been hospitalized several times during the past two months and again the previous week. Freda said she thought Ann had returned from the hospital before the weekend, but she hadn't seen her. Milton said he heard she was still in the hospital. Dorothy thought she heard the nurse say that Ann wasn't coming back. After lunch Freda made her way to Ann's room, where her son was packing photographs into a brown carton. Ann had died two days earlier.

In many nursing homes this kind of evasiveness and ambiguity is all too common and has a deleterious effect on residents. Most of us would find it intolerable to live in a place where we would not be told if a friend was dying or had died, or where a neighbor might disappear without explanation. Imagine what it would feel like to think that you yourself might disappear one day without anyone bothering to say anything. While many believe that this approach spares residents the pain of experiencing more loss, in reality it creates a confusion that is as insulting to these elders as it is to their deceased friend.

Residents often know that a fellow resident is dying – she has ceased leaving her room, the hospice nurse is on the scene, and visits by family members increase – and the chaplain should be an available, non-anxious presence to those who are aware. Certainly, residents who wish to say good-bye to a dying friend should be allowed to do so. In such circumstances, the chaplain can be available to help facilitate such visits, and help the visitor(s) process whatever emotions and thoughts arise. Though such visits may be "upsetting," most residents who visit a dying friend are glad they have been able to do this *mitzvah*. Some residents even share the vigil with family members of the person who is dying.

When a death occurs in a senior residential care facility, it is important to convey the news clearly and promptly to the immediate community. Recognition of this need has led some SRCs to develop standard protocols for announcing or posting death notices. In many Jewish homes, deaths are announced in the synagogue each week, but such an announcement may not be sufficient, as many residents do not attend synagogue, or may miss hearing the name even if they are in attendance. Thus, a resident from another floor or unit might be shocked to discover weeks later the reason why she hasn't seen her friend for such a long time.

There are a variety of print formats that announce the death of a resident. The one created at the Abramson Center has a dignified border, a graphic of a memorial lamp, and a simple text with four components: the words "We Remember," the name of the deceased resident, the years of birth and death, and a photograph. The photograph is essential because residents often have difficulty remembering names, even the names of people they see every day. "We Remember" notices usually are posted within 24 hours of the death and sometimes within just a few hours, after the deceased's loved ones have been informed.

In the aftermath of a death, chaplains should check in with staff and residents, especially tablemates and close neighbors of the deceased. If the chaplain is not present when a death occurs, it is important to check in with caregivers and with other residents as soon as possible, sharing the news with those who don't yet know, and with those who are not able to read the notice board. This check-in is an opportunity to listen attentively to their reactions, provide immediate acknowledgement that the loss is painful, and explore what this particular loss means to them, including what thoughts it raises about their own deaths.

Sharing Losses Through Memorial Services

For most of us the funeral or *shiva* (seven-day period of mourning) for a friend or loved one is an important opportunity to express and share our loss and grief, to give and receive comfort. In Judaism, attending a funeral is an expression of the high value of *kavod ha-met* (honoring the deceased); making a visit to mourners during *shiva* allows a person to perform the *mitzvah* of *nichum aveilim* (comforting mourners). However, when the death occurs in a nursing home or other senior care venue, the friends, neighbors, and caregivers of the deceased resident rarely have the opportunity to participate in these time-honored and powerful traditions. That is why it is important that other rituals be created to help them process their emotions and feelings. Periodic memorial services address this need. Some facilities hold annual, bi-annual, or quarterly memorial services to which family members and residents are invited. It should be noted, however, that a service of this type that is held many months after the death of a friend and neighbor may not really be a timely response to the personal sense of loss felt by residents and staff.

A better solution is to schedule a memorial service within thirty days of a resident's death, usually around the conclusion of *sheloshim* (the thirty-day period of mourning).[2] This is what is done at the Abramson Center. The service may be in memory of one resident or a few residents, but what is important is that it take place in the common area of the unit or household where the deceased lived, the place where their absence has been most keenly felt. In addition, posting notices of memorial services throughout the facility is essential so that other residents and staff will have the opportunity to attend services for residents they knew.

These memorial services follow the informal model of *shiva*, the mourning period that usually takes place in the home of the deceased or the mourner during the first seven days after the death. During the *shiva* period, people come together to offer comfort to the mourners, to honor the memory of the deceased, and to hold a prayer service for the recitation of the Mourners *Kaddish*. During memorial services in a nursing home, staff and residents have the opportunity to comfort each other in the shared experience of loss. When family members

---

2   Jewish mourning is divided into several periods of time: *Shiva* is a seven-day period after burial when the community traditionally comes to the house of a mourner to offer condolences; *Sheloshim* is the 30-day period, including *shiva,* during which all mourners continue to say the Mourners *Kaddish,* the memorial prayer for the deceased. Sons and daughters continue to say *Kaddish* for another ten months.

of the deceased attend these gatherings, residents and staff have the opportunity to reconnect with them and to perform the *mitzvah* of offering them comfort.

Setting up a sacred space to enhance this sacred moment – switching off the television, arranging chairs and wheelchairs in a way that facilitates spiritual connection, and turning on a memorial light – is essential to creating the right atmosphere. In addition, the chaplain might begin by humming a *niggun*, a soulful wordless melody, which sets the right mood and helps those gathered to feel more connected to each other in the moment. A reading such as chapter 3 of Ecclesiastes reminds everyone that there is "a time to live and a time to die," and thus provides an appropriate starting point for the chaplain to express the feelings and experience of the community:

"As people who live together 24/7 we share everything that life brings – the simchas *(happy occasions) and the sorrows. When a member of our community dies, we notice the absence, we acknowledge the loss, and we all feel more vulnerable. We come together today – residents, caregivers, and family members – to honor that person and to remember what was special about her."*

After commenting briefly on the individual's life journey, the chaplain encourages others to share a memory or say what they will miss. What emerges from the shared memories is a warm sense of the individual and a heightened awareness of how people touch the lives of others. Hearing reflections by other residents powerfully affirms that what we do in the last years, months, weeks, or days of our lives can make a difference: "She smiled at me every morning and I'll miss that." The affirmation resonates with other residents who, anticipating their own deaths, are comforted by the knowledge that "When my time comes, they will do this for me."

The reading of Psalm 23 should certainly be a staple of memorial services held in senior residential care facilities. It is a text that is familiar to most staff members and residents regardless of their faith tradition. More importantly, it expresses our yearning for God's presence as we gather "in the valley of the shadow of death." Concluding the service with the Jewish custom of reciting the Mourners *Kaddish* can provide opportunities for residents to bring to mind other personal losses, as well as to affirm their links with the past and hopes for the future.

Singing *Oseh Shalom* (the last line of the *Kaddish*) enhances the feeling of connection and being uplifted. As the service ends, there is a sense of peace and a heightened feeling of compassion that comes with our holding each other in acceptance of this ultimate truth.

When A Resident Sits Shiva

At age 96, Sarah was devastated when her son Fred came to the nursing home to tell her about the death of his older brother, Ben. Since Ben lived more than 1,000 miles away, Sarah had not known how ill he was. Fred told her that he would be leaving the next day for the funeral and shiva in Florida, but Sarah, who was in a wheelchair and dependent on oxygen, could not possibly make the trip. It was tragic enough to have lost her son, and the feeling that she couldn't even sit shiva for him deepened her feelings of despair. She felt utterly alone in her grief.

As older adults continue to age, it becomes more likely that they will experience the deaths of loved ones, even the death of a son or daughter. This is especially true of residents in senior care facilities. As mentioned above, when residents experience a loss, it is important to resist well-meaning desires to protect them from the full experience of grief. Whether or not they are able to attend a funeral, they need and deserve our support in observing whatever mourning rituals are meaningful to them, and in ways that are most comfortable for them.

When Sarah's son died, the chaplain understood that she needed to be able to respond as Jewish mourners do. Together they explored what was possible and came up with a plan. On the day of the funeral the chaplain and Sarah would perform the ritual of *kriah* (the tearing of a garment or a black ribbon on a pin), then read selected psalms and prayers that are typically included in a Jewish funeral service. During the *shiva* period there would be a daily service in Sarah's "household" so that she would be able to recite the Mourners *Kaddish*.

Because of the physical conditions and special circumstances of most residents in senior care facilities, holding a daily service in these facilities can be an enormous challenge.[3] Given the time needed for residents to complete their morning routines – getting up and dressed for

---

3 Some Jewish facilities provide services once or twice each day, and may have a dedicated synagogue for this purpose, in which case providing a *minyan* (the traditional quorum of 10) for mourners would be much easier.

the day, having breakfast, and receiving their medications – a morning service in a nursing home is usually very difficult to arrange, and in Sarah's situation was not possible. After dinner, most nursing home residents are ready to prepare for bed, so arranging for service in the evening may be difficult as well. Thus the best option was conduct a *Minchah* (afternoon) service which, according to Jewish tradition, can be recited any time from noon until sunset.

The service for Sarah's son was scheduled for 4:00 p.m., after naps and before dinner, a time when resident activities are finished for the day. The logistics, brevity, and simplicity of the service itself were factors to consider. Large print booklets were created, providing English and Hebrew options for the traditional prayers included in the *Minchah* service. A "*Shiva* Notice" was posted, stating that Sarah would be receiving condolences for the loss of her son from 3:00-5:00 each afternoon during the week of mourning, with a service at 4:00. Staff received a document entitled "What Caregivers Need to Know About Shiva," explaining the purpose of *shiva*, the meaning of specific rituals such as *kriah* and *Kaddish*, what to expect, and how to be helpful. Because some residents would probably need to be reminded about, and assisted to the service itself, staff support was essential to making the required prayer quorum of ten individuals (*minyan*) each day.

Sarah was deeply moved by the support of her caregivers, her friends, and even some residents she didn't know, or didn't remember. For many of the residents who attended, participating in comforting Sarah presented the ennobling opportunity to do a *mitzvah*, a sacred act of meaning and purpose. One resident in attendance was Jerry, a reclusive individual who often said he didn't feel worthy of attending the synagogue. However, when the chaplain asked him to help "make a *minyan*" for a woman who just lost her son, Jerry agreed to participate. As the chaplain steered his wheelchair over to Sarah's, he extended his hand to her and said, quite simply, "My name is Jerry, you probably don't know me, but I'm very sorry about your son." Sarah replied with equal simplicity. "Thank you for comforting me." It was a moment that elevated them both.

Funeral Needed

Mort and Ann, the nursing home's "sweethearts", were often seen riding side by side in their electric-powered wheelchairs. Both in their eighties, they had come to the home six years earlier when Ann's advancing Parkinson's

Disease made it impossible for her to continue caring for Mort, as she had for twenty years since his major stroke. Together they had participated in almost every aspect of life in the nursing home, and so his sudden death from a heart attack resonated deeply with residents and caregivers. Along with profound grief over the death of a wonderful man, there was deep affection and concern for Ann. Consequently, friends and caregivers alike expressed distress at the prospect that they might not be able to attend the funeral.

The situation around Mort's death attested to the need for holding a funeral service at the Abramson Center. The huge attendance and the accompanying outpouring of grief at Mort's passing also made it clear that the funeral was about much more than this one situation: it was about creating a sacred space into which residents and staff could bring their accumulated losses and deeply shared sense of mortality. Funerals held in a senior care facility affirm the beauty, compassion, and dignity of mere human beings trying to live as meaningfully and kindly as possible, even in the shadow of death. At the same time, the felt sense of being part of a community, both present and transcendent, is also a source of strength and joy.

The decision to conduct a funeral in a senior care facility, especially when the casket is present, requires a working partnership with a funeral director. It is also highly recommended that a policy be created, stating how frequently a funeral may be held on site, what happens if another event is already scheduled, and other logistical issues (e.g. parking for extra cars, charging a use fee if applicable, and who may serve as officiating clergy). In addition, a policy should clearly articulate the respective obligations and responsibilities of both the facility and the deceased's family.

Initially, concern was expressed about how many people would want to have funerals in our facility and whether the facility could accommodate all such requests. Fortunately, the concern was not borne out by experience. Most of the funerals that have taken place at the Abramson Center have been for long-time residents or those whose spouses were living there as well. Occasionally, a request for a funeral has been declined because previously-scheduled resident activities have taken priority.

In Jewish tradition, it is customary that mourners be served a "meal of consolation" upon their return from the cemetery. Some families, especially those who come from out of town, find it comforting and convenient to be able to return to the care facility after burial and partake of this meal, to which staff and residents can be invited. The meal can be "catered" by the in-house dining service or ordered from an approved outside caterer. It is also customary to have a pitcher of water and a towel outside the entrance for those returning from the cemetery.[4]

Embracing The Truth / Honoring Community

After the first funeral took place at the Abramson Center, a staff member made the following observation: "You would think that a funeral would make the residents feel too sad, but the strange thing is that it actually seemed to make everyone feel better – including me." It was clear that the event had caused them to experience "community" in a powerful and unexpected way, even as it helped them to mourn their losses in a larger, supportive context.

Conducting funerals and memorial services in senior residential care centers allows our oldest and frailest elders to experience ongoing and meaningful participation in a sacred community. In the midst of their own sorrow and vulnerability, they can find public validation for their grief as they engage in ennobling acts of honoring the dead and comforting mourners.

For many of us, attendance at a funeral stirs thoughts of our own death, and this is especially true of those who live in residential care venues. In the days following a funeral, or after attending a memorial service, many residents are motivated to talk more about what awaits them. Hopefully, out of their experience as part of a sacred caring community, their visions of their own deaths will include the hope that their community will also gather to honor them.

---

4   Washing one's hands upon leaving the cemetery is a symbolic act of purification from the spiritual impurity that occurs when one comes into direct contact with death. It is based on the biblical ritual found in Numbers 19:10-21.

Chapter 12
Promoting Spontaneous Prayer: The Blessings And The Challenges

Rabbi Gary J. Lavit, BCC

By its nature, formalized religion tends to standardize: one size fits all. Over the centuries, Jewish liturgical prayer was composed and formulated to cover comprehensive categories of human need. Categories, however, are not specific to the particular needs and experience of each individual, in his/her own moment of struggle. Yet, Jews have typically been taught to recite the words of the standardized *Siddur* (prayer book) almost exclusively, and to insert their own words or piggyback their own *kavanot* (spontaneous additions) onto the prayer text, at the most appropriate point within the text.

Alternatively, Jews familiar with the Book of Psalms have been taught to select a chapter from the Psalms which most closely approximates their current predicament, and to recite the *words* of that psalm with their own *kavanot* (i.e. to use the words of the psalmist rather than their own) to utilize the experiences of the psalmist for vicarious expression of their own struggles. Both of these methods of prayer require the individual worshiper to be familiar with the text and its meaning. The text comes first and foremost. The needs of the individual must be shaped to fit into the packaging or vehicle provided by the text. While valid for traditional Jews, many others find this approach to prayer to be a technical, academic exercise, not a genuine, heartfelt expression of and by the worshiper.

Many Jews equate praying with reciting words of a printed text; the possibility of extemporaneous prayer does not occur to them, and some believe that the tradition demands recitation *only* from fixed text and allows nothing else. As a consequence, many an observant Jew feels disempowered – even prohibited – from candidly expressing his/her true inner feelings to God, as if God only accepts mail submitted on the proper, authorized form. The Jew who says, "I don't know how to pray," usually means, "I never learned how to recite the Hebrew prayers." The elderly Jew who says, "I can't pray any more," may mean, "My eyesight has failed and I can't read the words." This misperceived insistence on praying only through the recitation of text, with the possible addition of a few personal *kavanot*, has resulted in spiritual disempowerment and disconnection for too many of our people.

An early biblical paradigm for prayer is the prayer of Hannah who, in her spiritual anguish, "poured out (her) soul before the Lord" (1 Samuel 1:15). For contemporary Jews, the experience of praying may be difficult or impossible, if one is required first to recite pages and pages of text, until reaching the point at which one's own words and feelings "may be inserted." Hannah was not encumbered by such a requirement, as it had not yet been invented in her time. She was able to express her true self, from the heart, without the intellectual overlays of law and literature later composed by the great masters.

Facilitated Spontaneous Prayer: Tailored To The Individual And The Moment

When praying with another person, chaplains enable that person to find expression of his/her true self. We listen and try to understand the life story, the struggles and fears of the person into whose presence we have entered. Then we try to put into words that which expresses the subjective truth of the patient's situation.

The first component of individualized spontaneous prayer is knowing the identity of the worshiper. In the standard liturgy of the traditional morning service, the essential identity of the community is affirmed with the words: "We are the people of Your covenant, the children of Abraham Your friend…" In addition to that which a person prays for, spontaneous non-liturgical prayer should also express the unique identity of the individual: his/her personal traits, character, deeds, values, relationships – as described the person or by others.

The structure of formal Jewish liturgical prayer dictates that words of praise and thanks first be expressed both before and after requests. These can be included as long as they do not contradict the patient's true feelings at the moment, nor interfere with the spontaneous flow of thoughts and feelings. Some elements of Jewish prayers that are familiar to most Jews may be helpful in crafting non-liturgical prayers, and might be included at the beginning of the prayer in order to transition from regular conversation and to engage participants in the activity of prayer.

Reciting familiar liturgical phrases can also help to connect participants to the Jewish tradition and to the community of the faithful at large. For example, the last three lines of the traditional end-of-life prayer *(Vidui)* could be recited in Hebrew as a conclusion to an otherwise spontaneous prayer at the bedside of a dying patient. While the main body of the prayer is spontaneous, the Hebrew conclusion with its familiar sounds would provide a sense of fulfillment at having "recited the prayer" for those who feel a need for such a formal recitation.

Although the focus here is on what the chaplain can do, from a Jewish perspective, anyone can create or facilitate individual, spontaneous prayer.

Guidelines For Creating Spontaneous Prayer[1]

What follows is an outline for how this can be accomplished effectively, followed by an illustration.

Gather background: One should be somewhat acquainted with the person(s) for whom, or on whose behalf, prayer is to be offered. Some elements of life-review are in order, with the following rules of thumb in mind:

When speaking with a caregiving elderly spouse, the question "How did the two of you meet?" may elicit stories of significance to the couple or family.

When speaking with adult children of an imminently dying parent, asking "What was it like growing up with him/her as a parent?" may elicit descriptions of personality traits and stories and with powerful memories – both pleasant and not-so-pleasant.

Don't be afraid of the unpleasant memories. Recalling feelings of guilt and/or regret can also energize the prayer and focus it in the direction of requesting forgiveness, or relieving spiritual suffering.

Ask a person near the end of life how he/she wishes to be

---

1   Prepared by the author for *Hiddur:The Center for Aging and Judaism,* Reconstructionist Rabbinical College, Wyncote, PA, for a workshop entitled "Spiritual Caring for the Family Caregiver," presented February 11, 2008, in Whippany, NJ; adapted and printed by permission of *Hiddur.*

remembered. Asking questions such as "How would you describe yourself?", "What kind of person are you?" or "What would you like people to remember about you?" can provide opportunities for closure and preparation for leaving this life. Similar questions can be asked of relatives of those who are unable to communicate.

It goes without saying that such invitations to share information and experiences can create important opportunities for the chaplain to facilitate more extensive pastoral care.

Request: The chaplain or pastoral visitor should be attuned to situations in which prayer might be helpful to the care recipient and/or family member. Note, however, that the offer should result from the need of the patient or family member to pray, not the visitor.

Ask: The chaplain or pastoral visitor should ask the care recipient and/or caregivers what specifically should be said to God – worries, concerns, requests, gratitude.

Draft/Preview: For the sake of clarity, the chaplain or pastoral visitor might offer to share the content of the intended prayer, before addressing it to God, "so that you might tell me if there's anything you'd like to add or delete or change."

Invitation: To nurture a more supportive atmosphere, others who are present at the time including nurses and doctors, can be invited to join in spirit and perhaps to interject their own words into the prayer. Those wishing not to participate can be invited simply to listen.

Since there is often structure even within Jewish "non-liturgical" prayer, such prayer might follow a format such as this one:

An *opening request* for God's focus upon us and the prayer that is about to be offered.

An *identification* of the person by name, with a description of his/her essential self, drawn from conversation during the initial gathering of information.

An *expression of appreciation* for opportunities and blessings received throughout the person's life.

A *description* of concerns followed by a *request*, also drawn from material shared in the visit or previous encounters.

An *expression of gratitude* to God for listening to our prayer.

If the individual is ill and is under the care of others, the prayer may include a request for God's blessings upon all who are caring for the person – both the healthcare professionals and family. For example, one might request that an overstressed caregiver find nurture and support from named friends, family-members, and the community of supporters. The chaplain or pastoral visitor might also pray for God's guidance and strength for him/herself in his/her efforts to provide effective spiritual support and comfort to the patient and family.

If the prayer is focusing on end-of-life issues, an appropriate request would be for God to reassure the dying person that loved-ones will find strength and peace, as well as a request for success of the caregivers in helping the patient to be comfortable until the end.

To be sure, while the above is a comprehensive inclusion of all the relevant elements, some might be omitted in the spontaneity of the moment.

An Illustration

What follows is an excerpt of conversation and prayer taken from the transcript of a pastoral visit in which this prayer modality was utilized. "Jake" was a terminally ill patient who was aware of his prognosis and suffering from physical pain. Always having seen himself as a big, strong man, Jake had trouble coping with being weak and dependent. He had chosen to forego further treatment, and expressed the wish to die. Family members had attempted to stop him from articulating his true wishes:

Chaplain (C): How do you feel about your life?
Patient (P): Enough!
C: You want to die?
P: Yes! God help me.
C: You want God's help to die?
P: Please.
C: You know it's alright to ask God to help you – to be comfortable and to die soon, without a lot of suffering. Maybe we should pray for that.
P: Yes.
C: Would you like me to try to put a prayer into words expressing your wishes, asking God for what you want?
P: Yes. Please.

C: Well, I'll try my best to pray.

P: Good!

C: God, here we are, Jake and me, right here. Please listen to us and hear our prayer. Jake is a strong man, and always has been, but he's having a tough time right now. Jake wants to thank You for all the blessings You've given him in life. But right now, life is terribly difficult for him. Please remember all the good things that Jake did and all the good things that he tried to do in his life. Please give him credit for all the good that he did, and tried to do. Please forgive him for his shortcomings and sins, because You know that we're only human and we can't be perfect. Now, God, please comfort Jake. He'd like You to bring his death about soon (P: Right.) and without too much suffering. (P: Please.) And please take good care of his family and those whom he loves, and give them good health and success in their lives (P: Yes, please.) and good thoughts and good memories of Jake. (P: Yes.) You are our God, and we turn to You and depend on You, and we thank You for our blessings.

> The Lord is God.
> Praised be the glory of His Kingdom forever and ever.
> Hear O Israel, the Lord is our God; the Lord is One.

These last three lines were recited, both in English and in Hebrew. The patient joined in reciting the last line – the *Shma* – which is familiar to almost every Jew; Jewish tradition encourages its recitation when death is near.

From the patient's multiple verbal interjections during the prayer, it is clear that he was an active participant. The prayer was not simply a creation of the chaplain. Instead, it was a prayer expressing the strong feelings and wishes of the man on whose behalf it was offered. The chaplain did not try to give the patient a pep talk or convince him that he should want to live. Indeed, imposing a prayer which would contradict the patient's true sentiments would not only have been futile, but would also deny the patient's right to have his own feelings and to express those feelings honestly to God. Indeed, the chaplain made no attempt to change the mind of the patient, but instead appropriately articulated the patient's wishes. Through the words of the prayer, he gave spiritual support to the suffering man, who only wished for a comfortable, natural death.

To be sure, the chaplain's response was within the parameters of Jewish law and tradition, which teaches that a person is not required to accept onerous treatment which extends longevity only for a short period – especially when the patient is suffering.[2]

Spontaneous Prayer Within Congregational Worship

In Jewish congregational settings, the words of prayer and the order in which prayers are said are of primary importance. In many a prayer group, attention is directed at counting the number of people for the *minyan* (quorum of 10), and in reciting the words correctly. Like the other *mitzvot* (commandments), prayer is an action, a behavior – something that we *do*. To those unfamiliar with the workings of Jewish prayer, it often appears as mostly a matter of proficiency in performance. Consequently, those who are not proficient or conversant with the prayer book often tend to sit passively while others recite or perform. In nursing homes or senior residential centers, those who sit passively may be most, if not many of those in attendance. Some may have once been able to find their way around a *siddur* (Jewish prayer book) but can no longer do so because of visual or cognitive deficits. Others may never have "learned how to pray" from the prayerbook in the first place. Still, it should be noted that many older Jews feel comfort in experiencing the sights and sounds of others *davening* (reciting the traditional prayers with the traditional melodies and gestures). Those with dementia are very often gratified to be a part of these experiences, and may remember – and begin to recite – prayers learned in early childhood.

Within the context of public worship, the chaplain's goal should be to engage the worshipers. Words and gestures, melodies and "choreography", all recited and performed, accomplish little if those in attendance feel disconnected and disengaged. Spontaneity that connects elderly worshipers to the service is far more valuable than *pro forma* religious compliance with procedural requirements. Spontaneous prayers also serve an important educational and spiritual purpose: they encourage elders to pray by expressing themselves "from the heart," rather than being stifled into passivity because they cannot pray "from the book."

---

2   Rabbi Moshe Feinstein, Responsa (in Hebrew) *Iggerot Moshe, Hoshen Mishpat II* (1985): responsum no. 73, sub-sections 1 & 5; no. 74, sub-section 2; no. 75, 1.

There are several ways to introduce spontaneous prayer into a more formal Jewish worship setting:

Our Own Prayer: During our Shabbat morning service in our center, when the moment is conducive (usually just after Torah Reading), I ask, "What is going on the world, that we want to talk to God about?" The question is asked in order to encourage participants to provide the ingredients for our prayer, in the style of a brainstorming session. I remind them that "This is 'our own' prayer, and it will express whatever is on our minds, right now, this morning." If there is little or no response, I will bring up an important current issue that may be affecting us as citizens (locally or nationally), Israel, or people in another part of the world. Then, I invite them to join me in spirit, "as I try my best to compose a prayer on behalf of all of us." I like to begin with a quotation from the Torah portion, the *Haftarah* (corresponding passage from the Prophets), or some Jewish text. Beyond that, the prayer is spontaneous. The subject matter of the day determines the content of the prayer. The opening text itself is instrumental, not determinative of what we choose to pray. There are times when no text presents itself as a beginning, or when the use of a text would be stretched or contrived. When that happens, the prayer is recited anyway. What is of prime importance is that those residents in attendance feel engaged in this prayer – that they have an authentic sense of ownership and authorship of it.

Yizkor without Books: A special memorial service (*Yizkor*) specifically to remember deceased relatives is recited four times a year in the synagogue. The usual structure of the service consists of reciting an introductory psalm, followed by a brief paragraph for each deceased person. The paragraphs printed in the prayer book are usually labeled: "For Father" "For Mother" "For a Man" "For a Woman." Each paragraph has a blank line, in the correct place, to be filled in orally (and silently) by the worshiper with the name of the person being remembered.

Frankly, it has always reminded me of a memo form: the wording of all the paragraphs is identical, except for masculine and feminine conjugation. The recitation of *Yizkor* appears like the verbal equivalent of filling out standard memo forms with the names of those whom we ask that God remember. Yet, worshipers are accustomed to this standardization. Unfortunately, the prayers often become a busy exercise of finding the page, reciting the correct paragraphs, remembering each name and inserting it in the paragraph where it belongs.

My approach to *Yizkor* is different: I endeavor to help residents – and others in attendance – experience this particular part of Jewish liturgy as something very special and very spiritual, rather than just a compulsive and rote recitation. First, I invite everyone to close their books. Rather than recite a selection, our discussions begins with the idea of having an immortal soul. We talk about the opportunities, difficulties and challenges that each person is given in this life; how our choices shape our souls – and how our effect upon others affects our own soul, which we must return to God when we leave this life. Other related ideas often arise: for example, in the afterlife there are no denial mechanisms. Each soul is cognizant of how well or poorly God regards them for the way they lived their lives. We hope that our loved ones did well enough in this life, so that their souls may feel God's love and appreciation of their efforts here. When we say *Yizkor*, we are asking God to focus His attention upon the souls of our loved ones, so that they may feel God's abiding love. This is followed by an invitation to envision their departed relatives:

"Now, think about your father. What kind of man was he? Did he provide for you? Did he give you a sense of security? Did you learn from him? Was he warm or distant? Who was he – honestly, with his strengths and weaknesses? How do you feel about him? (Pause) Now, in your own words, silently, ask God to remember your father and to let your father's soul know that you are remembering him now.

"Let us each pray to God silently. But for this first prayer, I will say my own prayer aloud, to help you find the words for your own prayer: God please remember my father. Please let his soul know that I remember him right now and that I appreciate him and miss him and still love him.

"Now, let's all be silent for each other. Now, ask God to remember your father and to let his soul know that you are remembering him right now."

Our attention then turns to remembering mothers: *"Now, think about your mother. When you were a child and stayed home from school because you were sick, how did she take care of you? When you were growing up, how did she raise you? When you were growing into adulthood, how did she relate to you? How did she relate to the other people in her life? (Pause) Now, ask God to remember her and to let her soul know how you feel about her and that you are remembering her right now."*

After remembering other loved ones including friends, we give our attention to anyone among us who has had the misfortune of losing a child. We might ask who they are and who they've lost. We offer our silent solidarity as they pray for the soul of a child or even a grandchild.

When the time for private remembering is concluded, either the cantor or I chant the traditional memorial prayer *Eil Malei Rahamim* (God, full of compassion...): first for those whom were personally remembered, then for Holocaust victims (including righteous gentiles), and finally for members of our US Armed Forces and the Israel Defense Forces who have fallen in battle.

This kind of *Yizkor* service fulfills our goal to engage residents as much and as fully as possible. Through their individual and personal prayers, those present are able to connect with God by raising up memories of the significant people in their lives. Through the traditional chant of the *Eil Malei Rahamim*, they also can feel connected with *klal Yisrael* – the historic and universal people of Israel.

Sensitivity To Disabilities

A classic Hasidic folktale tells of a small synagogue in Poland, in which all the men of the town had gathered for services on Yom Kippur (the Day of Atonement). However, there was one young boy who was unable to pray with the rest (perhaps we would understand him to have been developmentally or emotionally disabled). Nonetheless, moved by the fervor of the townspeople, he took out a tin whistle and blew it loud inside the synagogue. The congregants tried to silence him and force him out, but the rabbi chided them and said, "His prayer was the most sincere of any said here today."

In the world of senior care, we deal with people with many kinds of disabilities. At the same time we endeavor to promote a culture which helps and encourages such people to participate in any way they can.

Several years ago some of the male residents in our nursing home tried to assemble a traditional *minyan* and were concerned that there were only nine of the required ten men for the quorum. I happened to notice the absence of a particular man for whom attending services was important and meaningful. Just as I asked "Where is David?", a tenth man entered, and several voices answered my question: "We don't need him; we have a *minyan* (without him)."

David was a developmentally disabled resident who also had

dementia; he was also visually impaired and could not read the words. Sometimes he held his book upside down. But whenever he was in services, his face glowed. Although cognitively-impaired, in his soul he experienced himself as part of the congregation, connecting in his way with God. Even though there were a sufficient number of worshipers to conduct the service, I asked everyone to wait; I wanted David to be present so that he could have the same opportunity as the other residents to offer his prayers to God, according to his own particular abilities.

The Talmud teaches that "Merciful God requires the heart."[3] Moreover, prayer is called the "service of the heart," not mere lip service. God expects us to "have heart" – to respect and value each other and show compassion for one another. David's continued presence was testimony that our obligation to pray is not fulfilled simply by reciting the words; people authentically connect with God only when they are connected with each other as mutually respectful peers.

Spontaneous Prayer In Group Settings

Formal Jewish congregational worship occurrence is a hallmark in most Jewish senior care facilities, and thus introducing prayer that is spontaneous does not often go smoothly. When leading services in skilled nursing and assisted living settings, I have found it difficult to initiate opportunities for spontaneity during worship. Several factors seem to contribute to this phenomenon:

Jews raised in traditional environments tend to be more assertive about praying in ways to which they are more accustomed. Thus, any effort to alter the traditional service may be met with anger and resistance.

Residents with advanced dementia may recall traditional prayers from their youth, and respond favorably when they're recited or sung aloud. Their limited cognitive abilities may hinder their ability to respond to any changes in the liturgy, let alone offer prayers which are original and spontaneous.

Even residents who have been members of Reform congregations where liturgical creativity is encouraged may still not respond to such changes. They may still feel most comfortable with English readings from older editions of the Reform prayer books with which they are familiar.

---

3   Traditional paraphrase of *Sanhedrin 106b.*

And yet, there are moments in which spontaneous prayer can occur, as is seen from this example related by a colleague in another skilled nursing facility:

"Goldie" was 97 years old and had been a resident in skilled nursing facility for many years. Although she was unable to walk on her own, she was able to ambulate in a wheel chair. Every Shabbat morning, she would dress in a white outfit, and get herself to the synagogue for services. Unable to see very well, she simply sat in the back and listened to the prayers.

One Shabbat morning, Goldie surprised everyone when she moved herself to the front and approached the cantor leading services. "Please ask God to forgive me," she said. "I didn't light candles last night." Taken aback, the cantor, responded "Goldie, God forgives you."

But as the chaplain realized, more was required to address Goldie's spiritual pain. He wheeled her to the front of the synagogue, and opened the ark (the cabinet/closet which holds the Torah scrolls), and said to her, "Say what you feel in your heart." Goldie held the curtain and said, "Please, God, forgive me. I couldn't light candles last night because they broke. The nurses said they couldn't fix them before Shabbos began. It was the first time in 92 years that I didn't light candles. Please, God, forgive me." She held the curtain for a little longer, and then let go.

Goldie wasn't afraid to be spontaneous. Fortunately, the chaplain was astute enough to recognize the seriousness of the moment, and using his "priestly authority," he empowered her to pray for herself. One resident remarked later, "Today we were in the presence of true prayer. We don't get a chance to see it very often!"

Over the last several decades many Jews have felt permission to be more creative with prayers and to engage in spontaneity. Members of the "baby boom generation" may have been the first, but there are probably others including some who are already in their senior years. As more of them begin to move into senior residential care settings, a more open attitude to spontaneous prayers may be expected. At that point, the chaplain's task will be to find a happy balance – both liturgically and politically – between spontaneity and a more traditional format, while always promoting mutual respect among those who gather for prayer.[4]

The purpose of public worship is for a community of individuals,

---

4   Cf. Yevamot 62b, which reports extreme Divine displeasure at students not respecting each other.

representing the entire people of Israel, to collectively communicate with God.[5] For the community's prayers to be authentic and acceptable in God's eyes, the worshipers must truly *be* a community – not only in physical place, but in mutual respect and appreciation. By fostering ways in which worshipers can spontaneously express what is in their hearts and souls while addressing the Holy One, pastoral caregivers can enhance the experience of prayer for all.

---

5   Joseph B. Soloveitchik, "The Synagogue as an Institution and as an Idea," *Rabbi Joseph H. Lookstein Memorial Volume*, Leo Landman, ed., (New York: Ktav, 1980), pp. 321-39.

Chapter 13
Secular And Religious Jews

Rabbi Beverly Magidson

"Mom grew up on the Lower East Side of Manhattan, in a family that was strictly religious. They kept kosher, and she couldn't even go to the movies on Saturday afternoon. She'd sneak out once in a while, but if she was caught, Zeidy – that's my grandpa – would have spanked her. When she and my dad got married they no longer observed the Sabbath and holidays in the traditional way. After Zeidy died, they'd have a nice Friday night Sabbath dinner, but without all the prayers. They stopped keeping kosher when Bubbie (my grandma) died. They were already eating out in non-kosher restaurants by then. My Mom and Dad used Yiddish (both of their first languages) for secrets when we kids were little."

"We weren't really religious when I was growing up. Sure, we lived in a Jewish neighborhood, and my brother had a bar mitzvah. Mom would occasionally light Sabbath candles. We went to synagogue for High Holy Days and lit Hanukah candles at home. After my grandparents died our Passover Seders were a few prayers and a wonderful dinner. Mom belonged to Hadassah (the Women's Zionist Organization that supports Israel) – but then all her friends did that."

"I married Steve and we moved Upstate for jobs. We live in a suburb 20 miles north of Albany, so when Mom, now alone, needed skilled nursing care, I brought her up here. The Jewish facility is 20 miles away, but there's a nice, well-run facility right near me, and I could see her every day there. They have a chaplain and there are probably about four other Jewish residents. Mom doesn't keep kosher anymore, and she can come to me for Seders. It's worked out very well."

"But I sense something missing in her life. Yes, she misses Dad and the other relatives and friends. But she looks at the food – the tuna-noodle *casserole on Friday night; the sausage and eggs at breakfast – and feels far from her Jewish roots. At Passover time there's no matzah, and at Christmas time it seems like Christmas is everywhere. No one knows the Yiddish songs she used to sing for us. I can't find out who the other Jewish residents are, so she feels like she's the only one. She feels very isolated as a Jew. She misses her culture and she misses her people. The Activities Department celebrates Cinco de Mayo, Columbus Day and St. Patrick's Day, but no one seems to know much about Israel."*

I have heard stories like these over and over in my work with Jewish residents of long-term care facilities in Albany, NY and its surrounding suburbs. They illustrate a phenomenon in which an individual *seems* to have moved away from religious observance in a strict sense, yet still remains very connected to the *cultural* aspects of Judaism; ironically, these cultural aspects are strongly rooted in religious belief and practice. Nevertheless, when addressing the religious/spiritual needs of Jewish residents, professionals in long-term care facilities still may receive confusing messages about a particular resident's connection to Judaism. Questions may arise: Is the resident's connection rooted in religious belief, or secular but strongly cultural? And just *how* should the staff offer spiritual support that best meets the person where he/she is?

The answers to these questions are more complex than meets the eye. One can count many religious groups and faith communities in an increasingly diverse American community, and Judaism is certainly among them. From a strictly theological perspective, Judaism is a specific system of beliefs and practices that lead an individual to a relationship with God. Jews pray in places of worship (synagogues), and observe religious holiday rituals and customs as do the other religions of the world. At the same time, there is also a substantial *cultural* aspect to Judaism that enables Jews to be "non-religious", secular, and sometimes even anti-religious – but still Jewish! Indeed many people understand "being Jewish" in terms of an ethnicity, as one thinks of being Italian, Irish, or Russian. Music, food, colloquial expressions, and attitudes born out of the lives of Jews who immigrated from other lands may be non-religious in nature, yet still identifiably "Jewish".

In addition, there are significant differences between Judaism and Christianity that may make Judaism – both the religion and the culture – a bit harder to understand by non-Jews, yet are still important to be aware of, when it comes to working with Jewish long-term care residents. What follows are some rules of thumb and suggestions which hopefully will help long-term care staff in working with their Jewish residents.

Action Should Lead To Faith

Judaism's focus is on actions and behaviors rather than on specific beliefs. In other words, what a person *does* is more important than what a person believes. Sometimes the belief may be absent, or is so subconscious that the Jewish resident may be unaware of the depth of his/her actual faith. However, the actions that were taught to him/her as a child may be familiar and comfortable – and thus comforting – even if they are not accompanied by regular devotional prayer or affirmations of piety. For example, a Jewish woman may not actually believe that certain behaviors should be prohibited on the Sabbath as a day of rest. Yet that same woman may still want to light the Sabbath candles (even electric ones) on a Friday afternoon and recite the traditional blessing as well. This is because lighting the Sabbath candles is a ritual that her mother probably did every week at the beginning of the Sabbath, and she may have continued the tradition in her own home as well. Thus, even though a religious practice or ritual may be disconnected from its religious roots, it may still be a meaningful connection to a resident's past and to his/her identity as a Jew and as an individual.

A Vital Culture, Apart From Religious Practices

In most European communities, Jews were not part of the general culture. They spoke Yiddish (not Polish or Russian) or Ladino (using medieval Spanish) to one another, had separate schools, their own music, and their own foods. Many even dressed differently than the Christians around them. Some of this culture still exists independent of Judaism as a religion. Some Jews who came to America stopped believing in God; many stopped practicing Jewish rituals, but most still love the language, foods and music of their youth. Most seniors today were born in America, and yet they still enjoy the Old World culture practiced by their parents, aunts and uncles.

Jews Are Comforted By Others Like Themselves

Jewish residents may be embarrassed to ask non-Jewish staff, but they will ask pastoral visitors, "Are there other Jews here? I think I'm the only one!" When they come to a room with 3-4 others they are strengthened by being around others like themselves, and can be heard to say, "I didn't know YOU were Jewish, too!" Sometimes along with this is the discovery of shared family, friends, or acquaintances. The Jewish world is really a small community, and a Jewish resident is less lonely knowing he/she is still part of it. Another Jewish resident means there is someone who may share a history, a love of certain food, music or holidays. It means that there is someone to whom the resident can say a word in Yiddish, and not have to explain the entire context.

Orthodox, Conservative, And Reform

There are various levels of religious observance among Jews; however, most Jews in senior residences will identify themselves as belonging to one of three major religious movements in American Jewish life – Orthodox, Conservative, or Reform.

For the purpose of easy reference, Orthodox Jews are usually identified as the most traditionally observant, Conservative Jews are "middle of the road" and Reform Jews are the most liberal when it comes to religious practices. Within these broad groupings, one may find many variations of religious observance; these various approaches to Judaism make it possible for a Jew to be religious in many different ways. However, because Orthodox Judaism is usually identified as being the most religious, a resident may say, "I'm not really religious," but only mean "I'm not religious *in an Orthodox way*." In other words, they don't observe many of the traditional rituals associated with an Orthodox lifestyle. Nevertheless, many such Jews may still enjoy events that bring back special memories: a Passover Seder, or Hanukah candle-lighting, or even a traditional Friday night Shabbat dinner with chicken soup, roast chicken and other traditional foods (especially a *challah*).

Jews in the Conservative Movement may have joined their synagogue because it represented a convenient compromise between strict religious observance and a life-style more representative of mid-1950s America. Nonetheless, they enjoyed the traditional chanting of prayers and the adherence to traditions such as Shabbat (the Sabbath) and holidays among their synagogue's men's club, sisterhood, and youth groups.

For Jews who have identified with Reform Judaism and its emphasis on ethics and social action, traditional observances such as observing the dietary laws (keeping kosher) may hold little meaning, while staying involved in activities of social and political activism such as knitting blankets for a homeless shelter, reading for the blind, even writing letters to their Representative in Congress. The Reform Movement in the 1930s and 40s (when most of today's seniors grew up) taught that belief in God and ethical behavior are the heart of Judaism. Jews who grew up in Reform temples may see observing the dietary laws as unnecessary and archaic. Instead, many Jews found an expression of the ideal of God's gifts being available to all through social and political activism. For these Jewish residents, about an issue of social concern may be a connection to their religious roots.

It is also possible that residents may identify themselves as non-religious or cultural Jews without any connection to any of the religious movements. This stems from being raised at a time when secular organizations were actively organized in many American communities. Jews who once lived in Israel may simply identify themselves as Zionists.

Today, there are several other organized movements, such as Reconstructionist, Humanist, or non-denominational (sometimes called "post-denominational") Judaism. It is probable that some residents' families may belong to such groups, or that a visiting rabbi or youth group may come from such a synagogue. Many health-care chaplains are affiliated with the Reconstructionist movement.

Holidays

No matter how secular, most Jews will not celebrate Christmas or Easter, which celebrate events in the life and death of Jesus.

However, because the Christmas/Hanukah season has become very secularized in American culture, Jewish responses to it can vary greatly. It can be a difficult time for Jewish residents. It is important for staff to understand some basic differences between Christmas and Hanukah.

Hanukah is not the Jewish Christmas. Hanukah celebrates the victory of the ancient Maccabees over the Syrian Greeks and the subsequent survival of the Jewish religion and culture. Christmas celebrates the birth of Jesus, the founder of Christianity. Hanukah's unique message of religious freedom deserves respect on its own terms.

At Christmas/Hanukah time, Jews feel more different than at any other time of the year. Jews are accustomed to fitting in with popular American culture, but in December the popular culture celebrates an event that is religiously foreign to Jews. While the holiday has become more secular, its origin is still Christian.

Jews deal with Christmas in a wide variety of ways. Jews who come from Europe may have been persecuted for their religion there, and may still view any Christian practice negatively. American-born Jews have grown up accepting American popular culture (including Christmas) around them. Some even married non-Jews or have intermarried children.

Jewish residents may or may not want to participate in Christmas activities like decorating the tree, singing carols, or attending Christmas parties. Their response may be inconsistent as they try to establish boundaries.

Hanukah is a minor festival. Hanukah celebrations consist of lighting candles, *latke* (potato pancake) parties with family and friends, and gifts of small amounts of change (*Hanukah gelt*) for children who may use it to play *dreidel*. Major gift giving was unheard of until recently. Compared to Passover or the High Holy Days, Hanukah is a very modest holiday.

Many administrators and staff at non-Jewish facilities will want to respond to the cultural needs of secular Jewish residents. Even with limited resources, or in small Jewish communities, it is possible to do.

Help From The Local Community

If there is a local organized Jewish community, its members can be very helpful in serving the needs of Jewish residents.

For many Jews, a community connection has deep spiritual value. Their existential loneliness can be assuaged by the knowledge that the Jewish people – seen through their local community – cares enough to be there with them. There might be volunteers willing to visit, a synagogue or organization (like B'nai Brith or Hadassah) willing to do some outreach. If you have residents that have moved in from other areas, the local community may not be aware that they are there! The community can be accessed through the Jewish Federation, or a local synagogue, or Jewish Family Services. (Note, however, that a synagogue which identifies itself as Messianic is part of a Christian missionary organization. Involving its members or spiritual leader in Jewish activities will be counterproductive when serving elderly Jewish residents.)

There are some Jewish Federations that have materials that you can access about Jewish observances. There are also kits specifically created for long-term care facilities available for Shabbat, Passover and Hanukah at http://www.sacredseasons.org. Jewishfedny.org has a link to holiday newsletters with programmatic ideas and recipes.

Another source of information is Chabad Lubavitch. In recent years, this organization has developed an outreach program which provides education and support for elderly Jews in nursing homes and those who still live at home. Known for making trips to visit Jews in geographically remote areas, representatives of Chabad might even be willing to visit elderly Jews in towns and cities which may no longer have synagogues. The organization also publishes information about Jewish observance, available in print, email, and on their web site. More information can be found at http://www.lubavitch.com.[1]

Creating A Jewish Life

It's useful to have books with Jewish crafts, CD's and DVD's with Jewish themes. Yiddish music was a major staple of Jewish life in immigrant homes. Jewishmusic.com has a lot of good materials. Some of the best-known artists were Molly Picon, Saul Zim, Jan Peerce, and The Barry Sisters. The music and movie *Fiddler on the Roof* has wide appeal, as does the movie, *The Frisco Kid*.

A Jewish calendar can be a very helpful tool. Determining when Jewish holidays occur will avoid many possibly painful or embarrassing situations, even for residents who don't identify as religious Jews. For example, if someone doesn't want to eat or go to physical therapy on a day in mid- to late-September, it's probably because it's Yom Kippur (the Day of Atonement); residents many refuse to eat bread or cake during Passover. Consulting a Jewish calendar every month is a simple way of knowing what days will be important, even for non-practicing Jews. Calendars can usually be obtained from local synagogues or Jewish funeral chapels.

One way to reach secular Jews is through a social action project. They will find particular meaning in something that reaches out to the poor, needy, less fortunate.

Just as facilities strive to make meals attractive, they need to be aware of special food needs of ethnic groups in general. Our sense of who we are is affected by the food that we eat. Food is an important part of

---

1   It should be noted that representatives of Chabad Lubavitch are usually not trained chaplains; it may be necessary to alert them to clinical issues affecting residents' health and emotional well-being. Also, although Chabad Lubavitch is usually very accepting of Jews from diverse backgrounds, some residents may not be receptive to them.

Jews' lives, especially seniors. Supplying Jewish residents with Jewish ethnic foods will help them feel connected to their roots. The simplest Jewish foods may be available at a local supermarket (or a supermarket that is close to the Jewish community in your area): gefilte fish, matzah for Passover, a *challah* (braided Sabbath bread), frozen chopped liver, or frozen blintzes. Jewish cookbooks can be valuable resources for knowing what foods are eaten on which holidays. For example, blintzes are usually served at Shavuot, in the late spring, and honey cake in mid-September for the Jewish New Year.

Jews value community, and many find spiritual strength from just being in a community. When you bring Jewish residents together, they (and maybe their families) will create a Jewish community together. They may have their own suggestions for holiday celebrations, and may lead you to resources in the community. There is a traditional statement that "all Israel are responsible for one another," and that is a concept that has been accepted among even very secular Jews.

Awareness of unique Jewish needs shows sensitivity and caring. By creating Jewish culture and Jewish community, the spiritual needs of many Jews will be filled.

Chapter 14

Torah Study In Senior Residential Care

Rabbi David Glicksman

It (Torah) is a tree of life to all who hold fast to it, and whoever supports it is happy.[1]

Judaism teaches that the study of Torah[2] is a life-long endeavor. However, when one becomes old and frail, it can be more of a challenge as mental and cognitive faculties become less sharp. This essay is an attempt to describe how the commandment to be engaged in the study of Torah can be implemented in a population of Jews who find themselves in long-term care settings. While some of what will be presented in this essay is in the way of formal programs which are part of the therapeutic recreation schedule, there are other opportunities that may arise according to the specific circumstances of the residents themselves. A chaplain who is professionally trained to work with the elderly population and is knowledgeable in Torah texts can be most helpful in helping residents take advantage of these opportunities.

According to traditional Jewish belief, the relationship between the Jew and the Torah began when the children of Israel were standing at Mt. Sinai and received it from the Almighty through Moses our

---

1   Proverbs 3:18.

2   The word "Torah" in its limited sense refers to the Five Books of Moses, or the Pentateuch. In its broader sense, Torah refers to the oral interpretation which traditional Jews believe was also given on Mt. Sinai, which was committed to writing in various periods. A vast literature of interpretation, codes, responsa, etc. the study of which is also regarded as Torah study is also included in the term "Torah". Over time, Torah study has come to refer to the study of any writings that come under the wide umbrella of Torah.

prophet and teacher. Although a puzzling rabbinic teaching states that the Israelites were at first reticent to accept the Torah and G-d held the mountain over their heads like a barrel, the Torah itself states that they unequivocally accepted its teachings when they declared: *"Na'aseh V'nish'ma –* we will do, and we will obey."

This love affair with the Torah manifests itself in Jewish practice in many ways. Whenever the Torah scroll is taken out of the Ark in the synagogue, Jewish worshipers rise out of respect. Public reading of the Torah during religious communal worship is mandated by Jewish law, and when the Torah is read, it is read with precision and exactitude.

The study of Torah has always been an important activity in the religious life of a Jew. Since the Torah contains detailed information pertaining to observance of the *mitzvot*[3] or "commandments", it is natural that knowledge of the Torah is necessary in order to properly carry out the commandments. Indeed, the study of Torah is a *mitzvah* in the Torah in and of itself. Every day Jews declare in the *Shma* prayer *vedibarta bam* "you shall speak of them". We are mandated *"v'hagita bahem yomam valayla –* you shall meditate on them day and night".

After the destruction of the Temple in Jerusalem (70 CE), the Torah itself became the force which held the Jewish people together. As the Diaspora expanded and diversity in culture, language and nuances of custom among Jews became the norm, the Torah served as the binding force in Jewish life. Jews throughout history studied and revered the same books and commentaries, transmitting these teachings to the future generations. Various educational settings were developed in the Diaspora communities especially for this spiritual and intellectual activity. In modern times when Jews began to expand their intellectual horizons beyond the Torah, those Jews who abandoned their religious traditions transferred their love of learning to other disciplines.

Among the many references to the *mitzvah* of Torah study that are included in the rabbinic classic text *Pirkei Avot (Ethics of the Fathers,)* is a statement by Rabbi Judah the son of Tema that describes a lifelong curriculum of textual content and character development.

"He used to say: At five years the age is reached for the study of Bible, at ten for the study of Mishnah, at thirteen for the fulfillment of

---

3   *Mitzvah (sing.)* is normally understood to mean "good deed" which implies the voluntary carrying out of an optional behavior. The correct meaning of the term *Mitzvah* is commandment which implies that it emanates from G-d and is therefore required, not optional.

the commandments, at fifteen for the study of Talmud, at eighteen for marriage, at twenty for seeking a livelihood, at thirty for full strength, at forty for understanding, at fifty for giving counsel; at sixty a man attains old age, at seventy white old age, at eighty rare old age; at ninety he is bending over the grave; and at a hundred he is as if he were already dead and had passed away from the world."[4]

Rabbi Judah lived two thousand years ago and therefore his description of those who reach the age of ninety or a hundred years may not resonate at all with us. However, we can still derive from his words some wisdom that is meaningful and applicable to our contemporary lives. What we find in this Mishnah is a timeline in the acquiring of Torah knowledge and the development of character that is ever expanding as a person gets older. The terms "old age" (*Ziknah*), "white old age" (*Sevah*) and "rare old age" (*Gevurah*) are terms of respect indicating that individuals who have reached these stages of life are valuable members of society whose counsel can and should be sought. Furthermore, when the Mishnah states the ages at which various texts are to be pursued, it is not implying that the texts which were studied in earlier years are now to be abandoned. The pursuit of Torah study is developmental, incremental and lifelong. People who have reached the age of sixty, seventy, eighty and even beyond, should be engaged in all facets of Torah study to the best of their physical and mental capabilities and should be revered as resources for the younger generations in the community.

Our attention now turns to how residents in senior residential care facilities can be helped to continue to be a part of this important endeavor. What follows are descriptions of several programs that were introduced during my tenure as Director of Pastoral Care at the Central New Jersey Jewish Home for the Aged, now the Wilf Campus for Senior Living in Somerset, New Jersey.

At the outset, it should be noted that in developing and implementing formal programs in a senior care facility, and even when evaluating less formal activities, how "success" is measured needs to be reconsidered. In traditional educational settings, success is measured in terms of the internalization of a body of knowledge or the acquisition of desirable skills. However, in a senior residential care setting, with an elderly population, success must be determined differently. Since many residents have some short- or long-term memory impairment, "success"

---

4   *Ethics of the Fathers*, Chapter 5, Mishnah 24, Translated by Philip Birnbaum.

needs to be understood in terms of residents' immediate experiences. Thus, questions such as "What did they learn? What do they remember?" need to be replaced with those that ask:

> Are they participating in the program?
> Is it meaningful for them?
> Do they feel good about the program and being a part of it?
> Are they connected to their Jewishness as a result this program?
> Do these feelings remain with them once the program is over?"

If a learning program is based on learning a particular sacred text, the leader need not do exhaustive research of commentaries on the text (although such research might edify the leader). Instead, when preparing a program with the residents in mind, the leader should ask, "what does this text say to me, and how can I make this text meaningful for the residents who will be attending?"

Strongly related to Torah study programs in senior care centers is the place of other Jewish activities and programs in facilities where Jewish people reside. The former thrives in the soil of the latter. While Jewish activities are often a part of the therapeutic recreation program, the Jewish resident population should be thought of as a community itself, and Jewish programming as a part of their communal expression. On our campus, Jewish residents have their own synagogue, Hadassah chapter, library, store, etc. In addition to their religious importance, holiday celebrations are communal expressions and residents in particular facilities often develop their own unique traditions as to how Jewish holidays are celebrated. Formal programs of Torah study are often a special part of these community experiences.

The best and most appropriate opportunities to implement a program of study would be the creation of special "Torah Study" discussion groups to be held on Shabbat or holiday afternoons. Such programs should be part of an overall Shabbat or holiday schedule of activities including religious services, special refreshments provided after the service, the customary blessings offered at the meals (*Kiddish* and Grace After Meals), and any other specific rituals that are associated with a particular holiday.[5] Torah study discussion groups on Shabbat can focus on the Torah reading for the week or *Pirkei Avot* (Ethics of

---

5   For example, eating in the *Sukkah* during the *Sukkot* holiday, Passover Seders, etc.

the Fathers).[6] A discussion group held on a particular holiday can focus on a theme of that holiday. Texts chosen should evoke reflection and discussion, and when possible, should address concerns that pertain to this particular population – a goal that might take some creative thinking on the part of the leader. Teaching the text should not be the focus of the program, but rather a jumping off point with ample opportunities for residents to express their feelings and share their experiences and memories – which of course should be affirmed and validated.

One example of a Torah study program that can make a unique impact is the *Tikkun Yom Shavuot* or "Shavuot Torah vigil". *Shavuot* or the "Festival of Weeks" is a two-day holiday that occurs in May or the beginning of June and commemorates the giving of the Torah at Mt. Sinai. One way of celebrating this holiday is staying up all night engaged in a vigil of Torah study. Needless to say, staying up all night and studying Torah is not a viable option for residents of senior care facilities. Furthermore, it is probable that many if not most of our residents have never experienced this custom. However, by scheduling *Shavuot* Torah study vigil at a time more convenient for them – during the day or early evening – an opportunity is provided for them to connect with the *Shavuot* holiday and its emphasis on the experience of "receiving" the Torah in meaningful way. On the first day of the holiday the topic of discussion is customarily the Ten Commandments; on the second day the Book of Ruth is discussed.[7] Again, the focus of the discussion should be residents' memories, thoughts and religious associations: the goal is to keep them as participants in the celebration of the holiday, rather passive recipients.

Up until relatively recently, Jewish women did not receive the same level of Jewish education as their male counterparts. Since traditionally, a woman's religious role was focused on the home, her education was woefully minimal; a girl rarely if ever celebrated a Bat Mitzvah. In our center, a special program was designed in which a group of women prepared for their Bat Mitzvah. The curriculum consisted of practicing Hebrew reading from a primer, which included basic prayers from the

---

6   The text *Pirkei Avot* is traditionally read in the synagogue on Sabbath afternoon between Passover and *Shavuot* and is repeated during the summer.

7   The book of Ruth is read in the Synagogue on the second day of the Shavuot holiday, because it tells the story of the embracing of the Jewish religion by Ruth the Moabite daughter-in-law of Naomi. Like Ruth, all the children of Israel accepted Judaism on *Shavuot.*

liturgy. For those who already knew Hebrew, this was more of a review. Because letters and sounds form words and words form ideas, the reading practice was merely a point to begin a discussion ideas in Jewish religion, history and culture. After eight months, following the completion of the primer and many meaningful discussions on various topics, a date was chosen for the ceremony and celebration. The program itself consisted of the reading of the Ten Commandments in Hebrew and English and the recitation of a special Bat Mitzvah prayer by the Bat Mitzvah "girls". These were followed by a prayer of gratitude recited in unison by their family members. Each Bat Mitzvah received a certificate as well as a special gift. The highlight of the program was the Bat Mitzvah speeches which were composed by the residents. In order to help them do this more proficiently, one or more classes was devoted to learning how to write speeches. During these sessions, I would ask questions concerning such topics as their religious upbringing, education, participation in the Jewish community, meaning of celebration of Bat Mitzvah for them, etc. A tape recorder recorded both my questions and their answers. I would then listen to the tape and write down what each participant had said, and then organize their remarks into a coherent speech. Sometimes, additional private time was spent getting more material. The Bat Mitzvah program was repeated several times during my tenure, and was a joyous celebration for residents, families and staff. Most important it was an important opportunity for the participants to learn Torah.[8]

Ministering to a resident's personal religious need to study Torah study can often be challenging, but rewarding. When an elderly rabbi (whose family had unrealistically high expectations about his improvement) came in as a resident, his religious need to study Torah study was accommodated by setting up a table with religious tomes and a lamp for his use in the Synagogue. This created the ambiance of a traditional *beit midrash* (study hall). While he no longer had the cognitive ability to focus on abstract religious texts, he could at least look into books that had been sacred for him over the years.

A particularly poignant moment for me was meeting a new resident with severe dementia who had studied in a *yeshiva* (school for advanced

---

8   Editor's note: Similar programs creating Bar and Bat Mitzvah celebrations for residents in Jewish senior care facilities are becoming more common around the country. Our facility celebrated the Bat Mitzvah of seven women recently, the oldest being 94. The celebration drew 300 people and was reported both in the newspaper and on TV – CK.

Torah study) in his youth but had abandoned religious observance over the years. His daughter expressed that perhaps, he should resume attending the synagogue since he was nearing the end of his life. Staff brought him to the chapel for services on a daily basis, but he would just mumble in a mixture of Yiddish and English. One day I asked him if he had studied a particular tractate from the Talmud. He replied in Yiddish: "as a child". I then began to recite the text by heart and he continued to recite it. As a rabbi and as a chaplain, it was a particularly thrilling moment for me that I was able to open this door to his soul.

Many Jewish chaplains in senior care facilities provide the kind of religious programming described above. With these experiences also come similar moments of great joy and meaning. We do well to validate and affirm our own efforts in helping our Jewish residents retain their religious integrity and dignity. And there is no better, more effective way of doing this than by facilitating their study of Torah.

References

Carlson, Dosia, *Engaging in Ministry with Older Adults*, The Alban Institute, 1997.

Lumsden, D. Barry, ed., *The Older Adult as Learner: Aspects of Educational Gerontology*, Washington, Hemisphere Publishing Corporation, 1985.

Chapter 15
Technology To Enhance Religious Life

Rabbi James R. Michaels

The notion of technological innovation to enhance Jewish worship services might seem, to the casual observer, as a contradiction in terms. A Jewish religious service has a traditional format, is based on printed texts from the prayer book or from the Torah, and calls for recitation (either chanted or read) by those who are adept in synagogue skills. Where would there be room for technological innovation, even in an era when technology seems to change every other aspect of daily life?

In the world of Jewish aging services, however, technology is often employed to make the traditional *davenen* (praying) and more liberal services more accessible and enjoyable to residents. This chapter will explore some of the techniques Jewish chaplains have employed to enhance Jewish religious and cultural experiences in long-term care settings. In particular, a combination of low-, mid-, and high-tech innovations bring a new look to the age-old institution of Jewish prayer.

Customized Prayer Books

The most wide-spread use of technology is the creation of large-print prayer books. Almost every Jewish nursing home now has prayer books created expressly to suit the needs of its residents. Easily produced and inexpensive, this use of technology allows residents to use prayer books which are both light-weight and accessible to the vision impaired.

Davka Corporation has produced a series of CD-roms containing the texts for every service. All that is required to read these disks is a

Hebrew-English word processor such as *DavkaWriter*. The editor can find the texts he/she wants to include, copy them from the original, and import them into the new document. The font and size can be manipulated to fit the page, and to respond to the specific needs of the residents.

Once the Hebrew page is in place, the editor can type translations which are either creative or directly from the Hebrew. Chaplains desiring to create large-print books light enough to hold with arthritic hands could limit the document to a specific service, such as Friday evening or Saturday morning. Those wanting to create a service more to the tastes of Reform or Reconstructionist Judaism can select what they want, or even to create new prayers in both Hebrew and English.

Rabbi Sandra Katz, D. Min. chaplain at the Jewish Home of Rochester, NY, has used the *DavkaWriter* software to create an entire series of large-print worship services for weekdays, Shabbat, holidays and Days of Awe, as well as song sheets, Shabbat dinner booklets, and a Passover *Haggadah* (text of the Passover Seder). Rabbi Katz says that these custom-made prayer books promote resident satisfaction. She says she "starts where they are," with liturgies that look something like the books they have used in the past. Through step-by-step changes in the liturgies and consensus-building in the praying community, she aims to bridge denominational divides. In this way, she hopes to create community through shared prayer, even among those with differing religious affiliations. She says, "With the limited resources we have in a nursing home setting, and the limited support we can muster on weekends, I'd rather have one strong group than two weak ones."

Residents have selected a font that they find legible, and Rabbi Katz has consulted residents on service content, as well. During the worship experience, people with arthritic hands may have difficulty turning pages, so Rabbi Katz paginates the document carefully. With strategic placement of page breaks, residents are freed from turning pages in the middle of a paragraph. Using graphics can also regulate the page breaks and add aesthetic appeal, creating points of meditation.[1]

Another use of this same technique is the creation of Torah reading texts for each week. Rather than require residents to hold large

---

1   Editor's note: Along with using large-print, creating customized prayerbooks with spiral bindings and including residents' artwork to enhance the aesthetics makes them even more accessible to residents and adds to their sense of "ownership" of the prayerbooks themselves – CK.

Humashim (texts of the Torah with appropriate prophetic readings) with small print, they can hold a few stapled pages in their hands to follow the reading in either Hebrew or English.

PowerPoint Prayers

Rabbi Sara Paasche-Orlow, Director of Religious and Chaplaincy Services at Hebrew Senior Life in Boston, uses PowerPoint to enhance memorial services. Photos of those who are being memorialized are projected on one wall of the synagogue. She also is exploring the use of PowerPoint to project the prayers or Torah reading on a screen in large print for those who cannot hold the prayer book, or for whom the letters are too small.

Visual T'filah is a project of the Central Conference of American Rabbis designed to assist worshipers in finding new and deeper meaning through the use of contemporary technology. *VT* uses digital projectors and screens to display Jewish prayers intermingled with art and visual imagery. Because it makes Jewish worship more accessible to those with physical and/or cognitive impairments, and because it can be customized for a particular setting, it is an important resource for senior residential care settings which hold Jewish religious services.[2]

Rabbi Zev Schostak, director of Pastoral Care at the Gurwin Geriatric Center in Commack, NY, uses PowerPoint to enrich knowledge of Jewish holidays, customs and ceremonies, and current events in the Jewish community and in Israel. He says, "There are also many excellent professionally-produced videotapes (which may also be available in DVD format) that we use. Two of my favorites are Abba Eban's series on Israel, A *Nation Is Born* and the *Shalom Sesame* series which highlights the Jewish holidays."

Televised Services

Another innovation used with increasing frequency is closed circuit television. People in assisted living or skilled nursing facilities might want to participate in services, but may want or need to remain in their rooms, or in the day room on each unit. Televising services via closed circuit allows them to feel they're in services; it can be accomplished with relative ease and little expense. Most facilities utilize cable television with an in-house channel. All that is needed is a

---

2   More information can be obtained at http://www.ccarnet.org/vt.

camera in the synagogue with a microphone to transmit audio. Nursing staff would be asked to turn televisions in day rooms to the required channel, allowing the service to be viewed by many more people than would normally come to the actual service.

Although originally intended simply as a convenience, the use of television has brought unexpected benefits in several facilities:

Passover Seders: In the skilled nursing buildings of the Charles E. Smith Life Communities in Rockville, MD, we have used closed circuit television for several years. Because of space limitations or dietary needs, not all residents are able to attend the facility's Seders. Since the Seders are in the same hall as religious services, they, too, are televised. Residents on the units are given individual Seder plates and brought to the day rooms or their own rooms where they can participate in the rituals along with the leader whom they see on the TV screen.

One Pesach, the presence of a contagious intestinal virus required all residents in one building to remain on their units. In past years, that would have meant that the Seders would be canceled. Having the capacity to televise the Seders, however, allowed residents to enjoy what they otherwise would have missed. The leader sat – alone – in the hall and spoke directly to the camera. He said it felt strange to do so, but the residents said they enjoyed the experience.

An overflow service: Rabbi Sheila Segal, the former chaplain at the Abramson Geriatric Center in Philadelphia introduced televised Shabbat and festival services in her facility. Usually there is sufficient room in the Synagogue for those who come in person, while others are content to watch in their rooms. On the High Holidays, however, many more people want to attend than can be accommodated in the synagogue. Rather than turn them away, the staff sets up a large screen TV set in an adjacent assembly area (called the "Town Square"). She says some residents and families actually prefer being in the more open and less formal space but still be "in *shul*."

Options for Orthodox Jews: While most Jews have no compunction about watching television on Shabbat or holidays, Orthodox Jews will. This doesn't mean, however, that the technology is beyond their reach. Rabbi Zev Schostak doesn't broadcast live services on Shabbat or Yom Tov; however, he broadcasts his weekly talk "Rated 'R' for Rabbi" on closed circuit TV, as well as Friday afternoon Oneg Shabbat services. Many of these programs are also recorded on video tapes for residents who have VHS players in their rooms.

Televising Services From Synagogues

For several years, many congregations have made use of telephone technology to bring services to the home-bound. This idea has been extended to residents in long-term care. For example, for many years Rabbi Dvorah Jacobson, chaplain of the Jewish Geriatric Services in Longmeadow, MA, knew that a local Conservative synagogue had a telephone call-in line for members who could not attend services. Rabbi Jacobson regularly brought residents in Ruth's House, the facility's assisted living building, into a room where they would listen to the service.

Rabbi Jacobson has recently expanded on this concept. She became aware that Congregation Shirat Hayam, a Conservative synagogue in nearby Swampscott, had begun televising their Shabbat and holiday services via the Internet. She saw the potential for using this in Ruth's House. Working with the Information Technology department, she arranged for the "Movie Room" to be set up and equipped to receive and show the service each Shabbat and holiday. Residents were invited to come and watch the service.

During the High Holidays in 2010, the residents began making use of this innovation. Many of the residents went to the Movie Room and participated. (Rabbi Baruch HaLevi, Shirat Hayam's spiritual leader, had been notified that they would be watching. He acknowledged their "presence" from the pulpit, much to the excitement and delight of the residents in Ruth's House.) Although not as many people have watched the service on Shabbat mornings, a small group regularly gathers to do so. One resident who recently lost her husband says the Kaddish when it is recited by Rabbi HaLevi; even though she is not in the sanctuary, she says she considers it to be "the real thing."

Using Smart Phones And WiFi

Since 2009, Rabbi Len Lewy, a chaplain at Seasons Hospice and Palliative Care in West Allis, WI, has made use of smart phone technology. When visiting patients who are near the end of life, he contacts relatives who do not live nearby and gives them an opportunity to talk with their loved ones. He says that he always asks the patient's permission before making these calls, but 90% agree to it. Many times, if a patient requests a prayer, Rabbi Lewy will say it while the relatives are listening.

In addition to facilitating a needed visit, Rabbi Lewy says that hearing the conversation opens up pastoral opportunities, too. Knowing a relative's importance to the patient, Rabbi Lewy asks about the history of their relationship. Sometimes the patient will engage in life review while remembering his/her loved one; sometimes the patient and the relative will achieve resolution of a difficult or estranged relationship. If his visit ends with a prayer, Rabbi Lewy can include a reference to the relative.

Rabbi Lewy also says he uses a smart phone to store texts of various prayers and readings which he can use as needed. He also has downloaded songs and spiritual poetry which he can play for the patients.

In another use of mobile technology, Rabbi Zev Schostak has begun using WiFi to download various religious and cultural programs from the Internet. He stores these programs on his computer and uses them for weekly discussions. He also connects his computer to the Gurwin Geriatric Center's closed circuit TV system and makes downloaded programs available to residents who want to watch in their rooms.

Other Uses Of Technology

While tech-savvy chaplains and pastoral caregivers can creatively develop new ways to use cell phones and computers in their work, it's also advisable to follow the lead of family members who may have more experience or insight. A hospice chaplain once was called to a hospital to say final prayers for a dying patient. Most of the family had gathered, but one son was in Japan. A grandson, however, had set up his laptop computer in the room and contacted the son in Japan via Skype. The chaplain stood next to the patient, while the webcam focused on both. In this way, the son in Japan was just as present as the rest of the family.

In 2011, Rabbi Daniel Coleman, currently the Jewish chaplain at North Shore Hospital on Long Island, received a donation of thirty MP3 players. He plans to pre-load them with some of the meditations and guided imagery that is available via patient TV, as well as audio files/folders containing Jewish stories, music selection, and Torah lessons. Eventually, he would like to get sufficient funding to allow him to give the MP3s as gifts so that patients can use them to support their healing (and connection to community) beyond their hospital stay.

Other Innovations

Although the use of mid-tech techniques like customized prayer books, and high-tech innovations like PowerPoint and WiFi appeal to the imagination, low-tech can also be employed to enhance worship services. At the Charles E. Smith Life Communities, two different innovations have been employed.

An adjustable Torah-reading desk: After the synagogue had been redecorated, it was necessary to create a new Ark and *Shulchan* (Torah-reading desk). The older furniture, built in the 1940s, was both aesthetically unpleasant and impractical. The biggest problem was that residents in wheel chairs could not see or reach the Torah Scroll. How could they be accommodated while still allowing the Torah reader to be able to see the Torah text?

A solution was found in a device to raise and lower a table-top. The furniture designer suggested that it be installed in the new *Shulchan*. When residents in wheel chairs come to the desk, the entire top can be lowered so they can touch the scroll; if necessary, the top can be immediately raised for the convenience of the *baal korei* (Torah reader) and then lowered again when the resident would recite the blessing at the end of the *aliyah*. This mechanical device is available either in a hand-cranked or an electric version.

A light-weight Torah Scroll: Through the generosity of the owners of a local chain of supermarkets, the Communities commissioned a new Torah Scroll. The donors wanted to create a scroll which aging residents could carry, and possibly even lift. The original idea was to make a scroll which would have small dimensions, with parchment no more than 12 inches long.

When a local scribe was approached with idea, he proposed something different. He explained that, using the latest technological advances, he could create a larger scroll which could still be light in weight. The parchment would be thin, yet strong; the *atzei chayim* (wooden rollers) would be of light-weight wood.

The result was a scroll residents can easily grasp in their arms. It is big enough for them to know that they're holding an actual scroll, not a paper facsimile. When the scroll is taken from the ark, it is given to a resident in a wheel chair, who holds it while it is brought around the congregation for others to touch and kiss. Some residents even have sufficient arm strength to lift the scroll.

Looking Toward The Future

As long-term care continues to evolve, technology will probably play an increased role in serving seniors' religious needs. It's safe to assume that seniors and their families will opt for home-based care over institutions. Assuming they will be limited in their mobility, this will mean many more people in long-term care will be unable to go to services, even at nearby synagogues. Television and the Internet could be useful to meet their needs.

As the experience in Longmeadow, MA, demonstrates, the Internet could facilitate televising services to the home-bound. The technology already exists to transmit streaming video on an individual website. A small investment of capital would allow services from a designated facility (a nursing home or a local synagogue) to be transmitted to computers anywhere. People with Internet capacity in their homes could then receive and watch these services, either in real time, or at their leisure. This, in turn, could open up several other possibilities:

Local services: A local Jewish Federation, nursing facility, or department of service to the aging could televise services to the home-bound in their community. They would be able to watch services led by well-known community clergy.

Denominational options: National movements could provide televised services. This would allow people to choose Reform, Reconstructionist or Conservative services on Shabbat, and even Orthodox services during weekdays, watching the style of worship with which they are most comfortable. The Central Conference of American Rabbis (Reform) has recently made services and lectures available via the Internet.

Lectures and classes: Rabbis, cantors, or educators could present lectures and discussion groups during the week. If the presenters specialize in aging services, these classes could be tailored to the interests of the elderly.

It seems that a relatively small investment of capital on the local, regional, or national level would allow technology to bring religious services to people in long-term care, regardless of whether they are in institutions or in their own homes. The only limits to this would be the community's collective will and imagination, providing Jewish religious services for people in long-term care when it might be more significant for them than ever before.

Chapter 16
A Connection With Zion: Understanding Jews And Israel

Rabbi Beverly Magidson

In the memoir "My Life and Times," by Eve Wasser, who died at the age of 101 in May 2008, Eve wrote about her trips to Israel. Here is what she wrote in 1964, about her first trip there:

A small child's dream, an adolescent's vision, a mature person's hope and finally, realization! All of the above were steps in my life ever since I was a child of about eight years old. Until today – the day my husband and I boarded the plane at Kennedy Airport for a trip we shall long remember. A trip to the Holy Land – Israel!

Eve then tells the beginning of her dream, when her grandparents arrived there in 1914:

"It was then that my interest started. The yearning to go, to see the land described in our Bible, Jerusalem, where religion was born! As I grew older, my desire to go grew stronger. My mother often wrote letters to her family and in return received letters from them. Although each letter was filled with telling of their hardships, they also expressed the joy one felt of living in this land of lands. I often pestered my parents with the comment that I want to go to Palestine; not to live there, just to visit. To which my mother's reply would be: 'Some day my child, when you are grown and married, your husband will take you on a trip to the Holy Land. I may never see it, but I am sure you will.' … I never did stop hoping. I never did stop pestering. But in the last thirty-five years it was my husband with whom I talked and discussed this trip I wanted so very badly. So now you can understand with what emotions we kissed our children and grandchildren goodbye and boarded the plane for Israel. Here and now was the beginning of my dream, a dream come true after almost a half century of wishing and hoping."

Jewish residents in senior care facilities may not seem to be religious in the conventional sense of the word, but when the TV or radio news turns to news about Israel, their devotion to what is being broadcast often has a religious flavor ... and a religious fervor! While Jews may disagree among themselves regarding the policies of a particular Israeli administration in power, criticism of Israel by non-Jews may be interpreted (rightly or wrongly) as signs of anti-Semitism. Although American Jews are most definitely "American", still they have a special relationship with Israel. For many residents, their only trip abroad has been to Israel. It is not uncommon to see Israeli art objects or souvenirs decorating a resident's room. These may have been purchased on a personal trip there, or brought back by relatives or friends. And if asked about their source, a resident may respond with quite interesting stories, some told with great passion.

To understand the Jewish commitment to the modern State of Israel, it is useful to know a little Jewish history, specifically the historic Jewish ties to the *land* of Israel. Around the year 70 CE (the Common Era[1]), the Jews living in the land of Israel (or Judea, but called *Palestina/*Palestine by the Romans) rebelled against Rome. Rome defeated them, destroyed Jerusalem, and exiled much of the populace to different parts of their empire. For almost two millennia, Jews lived all over the globe. Much of this dispersion (Diaspora) was concentrated in Europe, where countries would invite Jews to settle in order to stimulate commerce. When their economies declined, Jews were often blamed for a wide variety of society's ills. What followed was often persecution, forced conversion to Christianity, or expulsion. Jews had no homeland of their own – only the hope of returning to their original place of origin, a dream reflected in the words "Next year in Jerusalem!" – a phrase which became part of Jewish liturgy. The hope of returning to the land of Israel was one of the motivations that kept Judaism alive during these millennia

---

1   The term Common Era (CE) is used by Jews to refer to the era more commonly referred to as "AD".

when the situation of the Jews themselves looked bleak.

The 19th and early 20th centuries saw the rise of nationalism throughout Europe. Small city-states and duchies were united to form larger, unified nations with single governments and languages. Jews began to think, "Why not us?" One Austrian journalist, Theodor Herzl, expressed this idea in a book entitled *The Jewish State*. In it, he proposed that Jews should have a homeland of their own, with their own government and language, and where they would be free from persecution. His idea gained a following, and in the year 1897, the First Zionist Congress[2] was held in Basel, Switzerland, to begin the process of creating a Jewish political state. While Herzl died only a few years later, the Zionist Congress continued the work of securing an independent Jewish homeland, preferably in the Holy Land of Israel. In 1917, at the end of World War I, the British government issued a statement called the Balfour Declaration, which supported the concept.

In the meantime, at the end of the 19th century, Jews mostly from Eastern Europe began to emigrate in large numbers. For years, they had endured intense persecution in the areas under Russian control. Most came to America and other Western countries, but some went to the land of Israel, where they found a small settlement of Jews who had maintained a presence all along. These "pioneers" developed the land, reclaimed swamps and deserts for farming, and built new cities.

Throughout the first half of the 20th century, Jews continued to come to the land of Israel, particularly in order to escape from Hitler's Germany. After World War I, the area known as Palestine – what is today Israel and Jordan – was under the control of Great Britain, which severely limited immigration of Jews. As a result, countless Jews could not escape Nazi persecution in Europe when they needed a safe haven. They could not obtain visas, and thus were trapped in Germany and in other countries the Nazis conquered. Eventually, six million European Jews died in what has been called "the Holocaust." For Jews, the question "how many might have escaped if immigration to British Palestine had been an option?" remains a haunting one to this day.

After World War II, the survivors of the Nazi concentration camps still could not enter Palestine legally. This all changed in 1948

---

2   "Zion" is the English form of the Hebrew word *Tsiyon*, the name of one of the hills in Jerusalem. "Zion" is also a synonym for Jerusalem in particular, as well as the entire land of Israel in general. A "Zionist" is a person who supports the idea of a Jewish homeland in that part of the world.

when the British left, and Israel declared its independence. For the first time in almost 2000 years there was a place where Jews could live without fear of persecution. It was hoped that the establishment of an independent State of Israel would solve the problems of persecution and discrimination that Jews around the world had encountered. Indeed, since its birth in 1948, Israel has absorbed Jewish refugees from Iraq, Turkey, Iran, Yemen, Morocco, Tunisia, Libya, Egypt, as well as the former Soviet Union. More recently, Jews have come from Ethiopia, Argentina and France. Israel remains the one place that a Jew is guaranteed a place of refuge. But the experience of the modern State of Israel has not been easy. Many of Israel's Arab neighbors have refused to accept her existence. In addition to several wars, Israel has also had to contend with, and respond to terrorism against her civilian population for most of her existence.

American Jews who have lived through this period of continued war and terrorism have strong feelings about Israel's existence. They may have family members who settled in Israel, either early in the 20th century as pioneers, or later as refugees or survivors of the Holocaust. Israel's story may remind them of their own efforts to bring relatives into the United States from Europe during the 1930s – a difficult task because of the Depression. And many Jews in America may have lived in Israel for a period of time.

Even before Israel's birth in 1948, many American Jews worked to raise money to build up the land of Israel and make it possible for Jews needing to live in safety to immigrate there. Many had charity boxes from the Jewish National Fund in their homes, into which they would put coins, in order to help buy land from Arab land-owners and to plant trees in the desert. They attended rallies calling upon the United States government to let Jewish refugees from the Nazis into this country, or the British government to let them into Palestine. Many American Jewish women still belong to Hadassah, the Women's Zionist Organization. In the 1930s Hadassah was instrumental in establishing orphanages in British Palestine for Jewish children who left Europe without their parents. Hadassah also built Hadassah Hospital, a major health care center near Jerusalem. Many elderly Jews still contribute to, or maintain life memberships in these organizations.

Thus, whether or not American Jews have actually have relatives living in Israel, they continue to have deep feelings of kinship to those Jews who live there. For many, commitment to Israel has become a substitute for religious belief. For others, Israel is seen as the only place where a Jew can live a full Jewish life, with secular culture and religious observance unified in everyday life. Israel's main language is Hebrew, and it follows the Jewish calendar in its community life. The main weekend day is Saturday, the Jewish Sabbath. Schools and businesses close for major Jewish Holy Days. Radio and television follow this rhythm of life. Street names and businesses use biblical names and names from Jewish history and lore. In the public schools, the Bible is the textbook for history, and stories about the ancient rabbis teach societal values. Religious and secular Jews alike build a Sukkah (harvest booth) for the holiday of Sukkot. When families gather for the Passover Seder, the story told may be the traditional story of the Israelites' exodus from Egypt or the modern story of Jewish liberation from Nazi persecution. When Israelis discuss public policy, they may cite rabbinic sayings in their arguments. Even non-religious Jews experience many religious influences in their daily life.

For many American Jews, Israel is a place to "charge one's Jewish batteries." Today there are many organized trips for high school and college-aged Jews. There also are tours of various adult groups, and many Jews have participated in such tours. One senior living facility, Cedar Village of Cincinnati, even organized a tour for residents a number of years ago and it has become a bi-annual trip. When American Jews visit Israel, they frequently speak afterward of feeling that they have "come home." In fact, some American Jews have "made *aliyah*" (the idiomatic expression for moving to Israel). All of this is important to know in order that staff will understand that when residents see or read news about Israel, they aren't simply observing events in some country overseas. Instead, their responses may be more emotional because of the deep personal connections felt by many of them, as well as religious attachments to the land they view as both a home and haven.

How can senior care facilities who serve Jewish residents continue to keep those batteries charged? One way is to encourage Jewish residents who have visited Israel to talk about their trips there, including showing any photographs or slides they may have taken. Reminiscence groups or travelogue programs with Israel as a topic would also be meaningful. If a resident or family members have slides of Israel, an "imaginary vacation" program might be planned for residents and staff alike.

Another way is to celebrate Israel Independence Day. Israeli music, food, and travel posters can help create a festive mood. Certainly seeking out resources of the local Jewish community for assistance would be useful; by coordinating celebrations with those of the larger Jewish community, residents will have a greater feeling of inclusion and connection to the larger Jewish community.

Weekly discussions of current events among residents will almost surely include reviewing the latest news from Israel and/or the Middle East. Staff or volunteers who lead these discussions should be aware of the sensitivity of Jewish residents to this topic, as well as their propensity to disagree with each other about what is best for Israelis!

The purpose of this chapter is to help those working with Jewish residents in senior residential care centers to understand the powerful connection that Jewish residents may have to Israel. At the same time, it must be acknowledged that the topic of Israel may very well raise complex political issues. Unfortunately, one of the side effects of the ongoing Arab-Israeli conflict and its accompanying issues is a stereotyping by each side of the other. Thus, if a facility has Muslim staff members, a proactive sensitivity training around this subject would be in order. The decades-old problems of the Middle East will not be resolved in our senior facilities, but at the very least, efforts should be made to create a modicum of tolerance and trust among Jews and Muslims, staff and residents.

Finally, it cannot be emphasized enough that while Jews in America are proud of Israel's accomplishments and feel strongly and deeply connected to her, they believe in America and are patriotic, active citizens. Most male residents (and some women) are veterans of America's wars (World War II or the Korean War) and are conscientious voters. "Next year in Jerusalem" may be the closing statement of the Passover Seder and Yom Kippur prayer services, but most American Jews view that as a spiritual goal for a time of peace and freedom for all, rather than a plan for moving to Israel. Indeed, they continue to be proud and patriotic citizens of this country, which has been a blessing to them.

Chapter 17
Cultural Competency In A Jewish-sponsored Senior Residential Care Setting

Susan C. Buchbinder, MSW

"The test of a people is how it behaves toward the old."
Rabbi Abraham Joshua Heschel

Excellent person-centered long-term care must focus not only on physical well-being, but also on the social, intellectual, emotional and spiritual well-being of each individual. This is a fundamental concept that we all, as care providers, strive to meet in our work on a day-to-day basis. Creating a culturally sensitive atmosphere is an important piece of this holistic approach to care. Providing meaningful cultural competency staff training in senior residential care settings can help meet this goal.

In a Jewish-sponsored organization, the mission and vision should be based on Jewish values. Jewish values must also be taken into account in the strategic planning process of the organization. Boards of Directors and leadership staff must have a clear understanding of the importance of these Jewish values and be purposeful in applying them in the workplace at all levels. Organizations which serve predominately Jewish residents have an obligation to educate their staff members – the majority of whom are not Jewish – about the basics of Jewish culture so that they can best meet the needs of the people they serve. At the same time, Jewish-sponsored organizations need to meet the cultural, spiritual and religious needs of the non-Jewish residents they serve, presenting additional staff development challenges.

Many questions arise as staff work to meet these goals: How do we educate all staff, whether Jewish or non-Jewish, about Judaism without sounding self-righteous or making them feel uncomfortable? How do we approach educating Jewish staff who come from diverse backgrounds or may have limited Jewish education? What is the best way to provide the necessary information without overwhelming an already overburdened work force? Faced with the many regulatory requirements for training in senior residential care settings, how do we elevate the importance of cultural competency education in our staff members' already busy schedules? How do we ensure that Jewish residents living in SRCs which are not Jewish auspices have their needs met? These are some of the challenges we may encounter as we work to meet the cultural, spiritual and religious needs of all of our residents.

CJE SeniorLife (CJE), a comprehensive nonprofit eldercare organization, supported in part by the Jewish Federation of Metropolitan Chicago, has implemented Jewish cultural education to give staff members the knowledge they need to provide the best holistic care possible for its predominantly Jewish clientele. This chapter will explore the challenges CJE experienced regarding the delivery of Jewish cultural education, as well as share techniques which were most effective in its senior residential care and other settings. Many of these methods may be adapted for use in other organizations.

CJE SeniorLife Background

CJE SeniorLife was established as a community-based eldercare organization by the Jewish Federation of Metropolitan Chicago in 1972 after the completion of an extensive needs study of the older Jewish population of Chicago. CJE began providing long-term care in 1981 with the opening of Lieberman Center for Health and Rehabilitation, a 240-bed skilled nursing facility. Sub-acute rehabilitative care supported by Medicare was added in 1997. According to its 2010 annual report, CJE currently serves over 18,000 clients, residents and families per year. The organization has more than 700 employees and a budget of over $50 million dollars. Community services provided by CJE include adult day care, home health care, in-home personal care, transportation services, home delivered meals, counseling and geriatric care management. In addition to long-term and short-term rehabilitation services offered at Lieberman Center, CJE's residential programs include a 160-unit assisted-living residence, with 125 traditional assisted-living apartments and 35 early to mid-stage residential dementia care beds. CJE also operates seven affordable or subsidized independent housing facilities. Funding to support this network of services comes from a variety of sources: approximately ten percent comes from the Jewish Federation of Metropolitan Chicago, with the remainder coming from a myriad of government programs, private grants, contributions and endowments.

The Importance Of Organizational Jewish Values As A Foundation

The foundation of any organization is its values. A solid base centered on Jewish values is essential to the establishment of a strong system of Jewish cultural education for staff. At CJE, this foundation is our mission, values and vision. The spring of 2004 saw the hiring of new organizational leadership at CJE, resulting in major cultural transformation and the beginning of a Board-driven strategic planning process. The organization's new mission, values and vision were adopted as part of the 2005 strategic plan.

As part of this transformation, the Board established a "Jewish Values Task Team," which later transitioned into a permanent Board committee. The committee established a new "Department of Religious Life" which was staffed, beginning in July 2004, by an administrator (this author). This newly created position was charged with conducting a full assessment of the religious and spiritual needs of CJE clients, residents and family members. One result of this assessment was the decision to hire a full-time rabbi who would also be a board certified chaplain, to provide pastoral care and religious leadership to the agency's staff and clientele at its various sites.

In the fall of 2004, the Jewish Values Committee was empowered by the Board of Directors to identify the Jewish Values of CJE SeniorLife. While the previous CJE mission statement included a commitment to Jewish values, it did not define those values. Through a year-long process of Judaic text study and intense discussion, the committee identified the five values upon which the organization would be based.

Commitment to these values and the implementation of the strategic plan has translated into on-going support for the Department of Religious Life on the part of its Leadership Group and the Board of Directors. Support has been both programmatic and financial. In 2005, a budget was established which gave the Department of Religious Life the resources it needed to provide quality staff education programming for Jewish culture. While there had been some informal Jewish cultural staff education prior to 2004, this was the first time in the history of CJE that the need for this type of education was formally recognized and supported with resources for both staff and improved programming.

Jewish Cultural Education At CJE SeniorLife

Prior to July 2004, Jewish cultural education for staff had been conducted informally. Historically, there had been a staff-driven "Jewish Dimensions" committee which distributed fact sheets about Jewish holidays a few times a year and periodically conducted Jewish cultural programs before major holidays. This committee had no established leadership and no budget. It was created to help meet staff-identified needs and was not well supported by the administration. The staff who served on the committee took on these responsibilities out of personal interest, but these tasks were not a formal part of their work responsibilities. By 2004, at the time of leadership transition, the Jewish Dimensions committee was no longer functioning. The distribution of holiday fact sheets continued due to the efforts of particular staff members, and a 45-minute module called "Understanding Jewish Culture" was produced for inclusion in CJE's new semi-monthly full-day staff orientation. This orientation used a 20-minute training film called "Jewish Life" produced by Baycrest Centre for Geriatric Care in Toronto, Ontario, and included additional information specific to CJE's programs and facilities.

In the fall of 2004, simultaneous to work beginning to identify CJE's Jewish values, a formal program of Jewish cultural staff education was also created. Sessions in the first year were conducted by the Department of Religious Life administrator for all levels of staff at Lieberman Center and other CJE locations. Based on written evaluations, these were received positively and with enthusiasm. In most cases presentations – which focused on the observance of High Holidays, Hanukah and Passover – were conducted as 30-40 minute formal in-service sessions using PowerPoint slides. All sessions included both lecture and participation from, and interaction with, participants. Distribution of the holiday fact sheets was also continued for both major and minor holidays.

The Department of Religious Life administrator also consulted regularly with Activities and Social Service staff, providing Jewish cultural information and resources to them as needed. In addition, a lending library of Judaic books, tapes, CDs and DVDs was established for staff use with the help of a small grant. Updates were also made to the Jewish Culture module included in CJE's New Staff Orientation.

Challenges

The second year of the Department of Religious Life saw the

hiring of a full-time rabbi/chaplain, along with the establishment of a formal departmental budget, including funding for staff education, and expansion of Jewish cultural education to include sessions on *kashrut*, (Jewish dietary laws) and Jewish practices surrounding death and mourning. The Religious Life administrator and the rabbi continued providing Judaic resources and direction for staff, including members of the Leadership Group, by answering questions and being a resource "checkpoint" for information.

Along with further departmental development, a number of significant challenges arose during the second year. While the sessions on Jewish holidays were well attended and well received at Lieberman Center in the first year, attendance dropped off dramatically in the second year. Analysis of written evaluations and discussions with key Lieberman staff identified the following reasons for the change:

- Limited staff time
- Competition with training required by regulatory bodies
- Sessions were repetitious for long-time staff
- Written fact sheets and formal in-service sessions were difficult for the many staff who were limited English speakers.

Other reasons included:

- A wide spectrum of current knowledge among staff
- Different staff positions needed different levels of knowledge
- Different staff members had different learning styles and formal in-service training was not necessarily the best way to meet all needs.

Successes

In order to gather information and ideas about how to address some of these issues, the Religious Life administrator began to meet with members of the newly formed CJE "Fun Committees." These committees, one at each major site location, were created by CJE's leadership team as a way to boost morale. Membership of each committee consisted of staff volunteers from a variety of departments and levels. They were empowered with a modest budget to create enjoyable programs and events for staff at their site. They became "advisors" to the administrator of the Department of Religious Life, offering insight into what approaches might work better in educating staff on Jewish culture. With their guidance and assistance, a more informal approach to Jewish cultural education for staff was implemented in the second year, and is revised each year as needs change.

One suggestion was to replace a formal in-service training at Lieberman Center for each major holiday – which required removing staff from the floors for 30-40 minutes – with a holiday information table set up the by Religious Life staff in the lobby where staff enter and leave the building. The table is set up at times when shifts change. It is staffed from 6:30 a.m. until 9 a.m. to accommodate the night shift as they leave, the day shift as they arrive, as well as the 8:30 a.m. – 5:00 p.m. employees. It is staffed again from 2:15 to 3:15 p.m. to reach the evening shift as they arrive.

The table hosts a display of ritual items and information about each holiday. Religious Life staff members distribute holiday fact sheets and are available to assist employees and answer questions. When the theme is the High Holidays, the rabbi is available to blow the *shofar* (ram's horn); for Hanukah *dreidel* games and a Hanukah *hanukiyah* (Hanukah candelabra) are set out; for Passover a sample Seder plate is set along with *matzah*, a cup of Elijah, and other Passover symbols.

Special foods are, of course, a very important element for most Jewish holidays. Free coffee is served at the morning table which is much appreciated by the employees, along with traditional treats specific to each holiday. Apples and honey or honey cake are served for the High Holidays, *latkes* (potato pancakes) for Hanukah, and *matzah* and macaroons for Passover.

In order to make the experience more "interactive", a word game or puzzle is offered for staff to complete, with the answers to be found in the holiday fact sheet or other visual materials provided on the table. Employees are encouraged to work together to complete the puzzles and to engage Department of Religious Life staff for assistance, which often leads to many questions being answered informally. Once completed, these puzzles become each staff person's entry in a drawing for small prizes, thus providing incentive for their completion.

In 2010, a series of holiday display boards were created by a summer intern assigned to the Religious Life department to enhance the information tables. Each board presents basic information about a holiday and photographs of various ritual items using PowerPoint slides which are printed, laminated and mounted on tri-fold heavy duty display boards which are available at office supply stores. Visual displays of this sort can be very effective in reaching staff who have little time or who may lack sufficient English skills to read the holiday fact sheets. The colorful and attractive photos and graphics on the boards help draw people to the table. These boards have also been displayed in our business office as a way to disseminate Jewish cultural information to staff who are based there. In addition, display boards about common Jewish symbols and about famous Jewish figures in sports, entertainment, science and the arts were also created by the intern and have been used as educational displays for both staff and residents in various locations.

The information table format has had obvious benefits:

- It creates a way for staff members to participate in an informal enjoyable activity, rather than a formal in-service in a classroom setting.
- It is less time-consuming for staff and does not take them off the floors.
- It has also enabled Religious Life staff to reach virtually all of the Lieberman employees, which was not possible using the previous format.

The new format also has allowed employees who might not speak up in a classroom situation to ask questions in a more personal setting and has allowed for more interaction with their peers, sometimes resulting in more experienced staff assisting co-workers in finding answers to puzzle questions. It also accommodates the varied learning styles and levels of knowledge represented among staff members. While some tend to learn better through visual displays and actually handling the ritual items on the table, others learn better through written words and cognitive tasks. Those who already have some knowledge are able to ask more in-depth questions in an informal way, rather than in front of a class. Those who know less are able to become acquainted with "the basics" without being overwhelmed with too much information.

Another example of our informal approach to staff training in Jewish culture was a Kosher Food Fair that was conducted for CJE's business office staff. While the employees in our residential settings have a lot of exposure to kosher food and the rules of *kashrut* as they serve meals to residents, many in our business office sometimes have difficulty understanding the organization's commitment to providing only kosher food at staff functions, meetings and events even though the majority of participants may not "keep kosher", much less be Jewish.

In order to educate staff, the Department of Religious Life and the Fun Committee sponsored a Kosher Food Fair offering many examples of packaged and prepared foods which just happen to be kosher, and which any shopper might find in the grocery store. In order to help staff recognize what food products are certifiably "kosher", a "*hechsher* (kosher certification symbol) hunt" was included as part of the Fair. Participants were given "bingo" style cards with different *hechshers* in each square. As they circulated from table to table tasting the kosher treats, they examined food packaging for the different *hechshers*, indicating on their card which products contained each *hechsher*. Information displays about the basics of *kashrut* were located at each "station." Again, upon completion of the cards, staff members could submit them as entries in prize drawings. This exercise became an essential tool to help staff members who were responsible for buying refreshments for staff events and meetings. The exercise also helped to "de-mystify" the rules of *kashrut* and allowed staff to see the dietary laws as a normal part of Jewish life instead of as a restrictive burden.

These are some examples of the various creative approaches to cultural education which have worked at CJE. To be sure, smaller facilities may not have the resources to facilitate programs such as the ones described above, particularly in regard to space availability or funding for refreshments and game prizes. In some settings, alternative modes, such as a learning "cart," displaying ritual items and offering small culinary treats which can be brought around to staff, might accomplish similar goals.

Concluding "Key" Ideas

At CJE SeniorLife, informal, interactive, and entertaining programs have proved to be more successful in educating staff about Jewish culture than formal in-service trainings. It is key that sessions and programs be scheduled at convenient times for employees who work very hard and have grueling schedules. Instead of expecting staff to come to the cultural education program, it is key to bring the program to the staff: sessions and programs should be scheduled in locations where staff members naturally congregate, as well as near entrances to facilities, in order "catch them" when they are coming in or leaving. It is key that program planners be flexible and willing to make changes and experiment with new ideas. Finally, it is key to involve staff members in the planning and implementation of these programs, when possible, to ensure the quality and success of the programs themselves. Providing quality Jewish cultural education for staff in senior residential care facilities where Jewish people live takes serious programmatic and financial support from administrators and managers. Along with the courage to experiment and persistence in trying new approaches, creative thinking, collaboration, and the willingness to listen carefully to and involve the staff members with whom we work will certainly lead to a Jewish cultural competency program with which all staff will resonate.

But when all else fails ... food always helps!

Resources

Training Films and Materials
"Jewish Life": Film and companion booklet, Baycrest Centre for Geriatric Care, Toronto, Ontario. www.baycrest.org

"The Art of Jewish Caregiving": Films and companion booklet, Jewish Home and Aging Services, Detroit, Michigan. www.jhas.org

Books
The Jewish Catalog, Siegal, Strassfeld & Strassfeld
The Jewish Holidays, Michael Strassfeld
The Jewish Year, Barbara Rush

Websites
www.MyJewishLearning.org
Information, articles, materials and quizzes presented from different Jewish perspectives and great on-line newsletters.
www.sacredseasons.org
Sacred Seasons Celebration Kits which help staff with limited Jewish knowledge provide Jewish holiday programming for their Jewish residents. Produced by Hiddur, a program of the Reconstructionist Rabbinical College.

Puzzle-Making Websites
www.discoveryeducation.com
www.armoredpenguin.com
www.puzzle-maker.com

CJE SeniorLife Mission And Values

The mission of CJE SeniorLife is to facilitate independence of older adults and to enhance quality of life by advocating on their behalf and by offering programs and services throughout the continuum of care for individuals, families and the community.

At CJE SeniorLife, we fulfill our mission and realize our vision for and on behalf of our Clients, our Clients' families, our Staff, our Board Members, and our Volunteers by striving for excellence through Respect, Advocacy, Compassion, Intention and Accountability.

- *Respect / Kavod*
  "Rise in the presence of age and show deference to the old."
  Leviticus 19:32

We recognize, honor, and acknowledge the inherent value of each person for their wisdom, their culture, their background, and their unique history.

- *Advocacy / Timicha*
  "Learn to do well, seek justices, relieve the oppressed."
  Isaiah 1:17

We give voice to our clients' needs and facilitate positive action on their behalf. Furthermore, we encourage public policy and continuously educate ourselves and the community to benefit our clients.

- *Compassion / Chesed*
  "Have compassion and mercy for one another."
  Zachariah 7:9

We treat everyone with caring, sensitivity, understanding, and supportive responsiveness.

- *Intention / Kavanah*
  "Whatever your hand finds to do, do it with all your might."
  Ecclesiastes 9:10

We approach our work and each task with mindful consideration as to what we are doing and why we are doing it, as individuals and as an Agency.

- *Accountability / Arevut*
  "We are all held accountable to one another."
  Adapted from Babylonian Talmud
  Shavuot 39a.

We are responsible individually and as an Agency for honest, accurate work and interaction with others. We plan strategically and provide measurable quality care with clear fiscal and ethical responsibility.

CJE SeniorLife Vision Statement

CJE SeniorLife will be recognized as the leading provider of programs and services for older adults, responsive to changing community needs throughout the continuum of care.

CJE SeniorLife is dedicated to collaborating with the Jewish Federation of Metropolitan Chicago, hospitals and the larger medical community, other older adult organizations, government agencies, funders and other community organizations. Our work will be enhanced though grants, research and public policy activities. By continually evaluating and improving our operations, CJE SeniorLife will be fiscally sound with balanced social and economic objectives.

CJE SeniorLife is committed to attracting, retaining and developing management, staff, Board members and volunteers who are engaged in fulfilling our mission.

CJE SeniorLife will strive to be the preferred provider for the Jewish community of metropolitan Chicago.

CJE SeniorLife is a partner in serving our community, supported by the Jewish United Fund/Jewish Federation of Metropolitan Chicago.

Chapter 18
Lessons Of A Lifetime: Creating Ethical Wills In Senior Residential Care Settings

Joshua M. Z. Stanton and Hedy Peyser

From the moment we emerge from the womb, we embark on a life journey of personal growth – physically, emotionally, spiritually. In addition to experiencing changes in our bodies, we experience changes in our psyches and our souls – changes caused by important moments in life that make us who we are. Birth, time with one's family, early education, graduation, marriage, children, the death of loved ones, career transitions – indeed, all of the living that goes on between each occasion – contribute to the personal development we all continuously undergo until our inevitable end.

Yet, the cessation of personal growth – if only apparent – may in fact contribute to the angst, pain, and regret that too often accompanies "getting older." This cessation often results in individuals not taking the time and opportunity to reflect back on their lives, as their lives are concluding. A feeling of disempowerment may result and prove to be an undesirable yet prominent part of a person's final weeks, months, and even years.

Grappling with existential questions at the end of one's life, Jewish older adults in particular may experience this disempowerment, which is often aggravated by a sense of despair and fear. This may be due to the fact that many Jewish older adults, products of the secular culture in which they were raised, were not taught to believe in the traditional Jewish teaching that there IS a life after death – a tenet which affords a certain hope that often mitigates this despair and fear.[1]

---

1   Although there is no official rabbinic "dogma" on what exactly happens after death, Judaism has affirmed a belief in an afterlife for the last

By contrast, it is far more uniformly recognized among all Jews that Judaism's tradition of honoring the elderly deems the later years as a time for introspection and reflection. For centuries, if not millennia, Jewish elders have taken advantage of that time by recording what are called "ethical wills" – statements of personal values to be bequeathed to families and loved ones. Rather than providing a material bequest, an ethical will transmits a moral and spiritual legacy containing an individual's summary of what he/she has learned from life – hopes and dreams as well as regrets and sorrows – to be passed on to those who will come after. Because their content offers a tangible "bit of immortality", ethical wills may be a useful means by which to provide effective pastoral care: by providing a forum for expressing feelings about the life that a person has lived, an ethical will can be a vehicle for gaining insight and displaying creativity towards the end of one's life. It can also provide an ideal opportunity for older adults to continue their journeys of personal growth through the process of introspection and the drawing together of life's experiences into a single document.

Appreciating The History Of Ethical Wills

The beauty of ethical wills is found not only in their form, but also in their history. They date back to biblical times. An early example of an ethical will is Jacob's addressing his children and expressing his hopes for each one of them, as is recorded in the book of Genesis, chapter 49.2. Unlike oral histories, which are supposed to objectively chronicle a person's life experiences, ethical wills convey what a person has learned from those experiences. In earlier times, what was learned and shared was transmitted orally from generation to generation. However, by the 12th century, ethical wills had evolved into written statements of values

---

two millennia. Cf. Simcha Paull Raphael's *Jewish Views of the Afterlife* and Neil Gillman's *The Death of Death*. Editors' note: Exploring the reasons for the discrepancy between Jewish teachings and what individual Jews believe is beyond the scope of this chapter. Significantly, one indication of the lack of uniformity of beliefs and attitudes on this subject is evidenced by the views of one of the authors of this chapter (Joshua Stanton), which substantially diverge from more traditional ones. For a more focused discussion on this discrepancy, cf. Rabbi Bev Magidson's chapter, "Secular and Religious Jews".

2   Cf. Israel Abrahams. Introduction. *Hebrew Ethical Wills*. Philadelphia: JPS, 1976: page xix.

that could be more reliably conveyed than their oral predecessors.[3] And while these documents became particularly prevalent within Jewish communities, they are also known to have been extant within Christian and Muslim communities. As Israel Abrahams notes in his classic analysis of these documents, *Hebrew Ethical Wills*:

> ...the ethical testament has a long and continuous history in Jewish literature. That literature did not monopolize the genre. The Arabs held the ethical will (included under the general title *Wasaya*) in such high esteem that they would ascribe documents of the kind to the reverend sages like *Lokman*. In Christian circles, too, we find similar phenomena.[4]

With a long and revered presence in all three Abrahamic religions, ethical wills have reemerged in recent years as a way to ensure that the values and wisdom of one generation are conveyed to the next, with the hope that future generations will thereby lead better, more fulfilling lives.[5] Significantly, a recent pilot study has linked the creation of ethical wills to a reduction in the suffering of cancer patients.[6] One of its conclusions suggests that a perceived "loss of meaning" and an ongoing concern for loved ones may contribute to a cancer patient's overall discomfort.

It is therefore curious that, as an aid to help older adults cope with the challenges of aging and frailty, ethical wills are an under-utilized resource. Despite their lengthy history, inherent value, and potential medical applications, there are often challenges that impede residents in senior care facilities from creating them. Many residents in these facilities simply lack the physical capacity to write down their thoughts or record them in other ways. And even for those who do possess the ability and the desire, the process can be emotionally daunting.

For these individuals, some of their most profound or life-changing experiences may also have been their least pleasant – and recounting

---

3   Ibid.

4   Ibid., page xxii.

5   A lull in their use appears to have occurred in the West following the Renaissance.

6   Cf. Charles E. Gessert, Barry K. Baines, Steven A. Kuross, Cinda Clark, and Irina V. Haller. "Ethical Wills and Suffering in Patients with Cancer," *Journal of Palliative Medicine*, Volume 7, Number 4, August, 2004.

them may bring back emotions long since buried which they would prefer to keep buried, particularly if they are writing alone. Others may not know how or where to begin: should they talk about their childhood? Is it appropriate to start with a small vignette? To be sure, some of these impediments (e.g. dealing with difficult memories) may be unavoidable. But all of them are certainly manageable, especially when a supportive context is provided in which individuals can do their own reflecting and writing.

In March 2006, we founded *Lessons of a Lifetime: The Ethical Will Project of the Hebrew Home*[7] to encourage residents of the Charles E. Smith Life Communities in Rockville, Maryland, to do just that. Though there are aspects of the project that are unique to the Charles E. Smith community, many aspects of the program can be readily be duplicated and implemented by pastoral caregivers and other senior residential care staff around the country.[8]

Initiating the process rests on the introduction of twenty-two thought-provoking questions to participants, designed to help them recall the most significant moments in their lives and reflect on their meaning. These "22 Questions for Ethical Wills©" are divided into eight categories:

- Values and education
- Formative thoughts and beliefs
- Words of wisdom
- Life experiences
- Life's lessons
- Regrets and gratitude
- Key Decisions
- Change and the future

We found that providing a template of this sort better facilitates the process of writing an ethical will by providing a focused direction and guidance, rather than forcing the writer to search for the right questions to both ask and answer. It is, however, designed to be flexible,

---

7   Registered trademark, all rights reserved.

8   For more information about how to start a similar program at your senior residence, or if you are interested in using our program materials, see the "Ethical Wills" section of http://www.hebrew-home.org/site/ PageServer?pagename=family.

since certain questions will engage some people more than others. In addition, participants are encouraged to skip any questions that may cause them mental or emotional distress, and also to expand upon those to which they particularly relate.

From Thoughtful Questions To Intergenerational Initiative

Of course, answering a set of questions alone is hardly sufficient to ensure that an individual will be able to compose an ethical will. Participants – especially those who have physical limitations – may need assistance from others to interview them and do the actual crafting of the ethical will from the participants' responses. In many instances, a chaplain or other pastoral care provider is ideal for this task. However, due to the work being quite "labor intensive" and the fact that many senior residential care facilities may have at most one chaplain/pastoral caregiver on staff, making such a project the sole responsibility of this individual is most often not practical – which is why creating a program to train volunteers to work with residents is much more feasible. Besides making the project more time-efficient, it affords opportunities for both volunteers and resident participants to forge new and mutually meaningful friendships.

Our program, *Lessons of a Lifetime*, pairs each resident participant with a student volunteer (volunteers range from 12 to 25 years of age), each of whom has been given special training in the techniques for creating and recording ethical wills. From what we have seen, these intergenerational partnerships have indeed proven beneficial to both the students and the participants. Students have the opportunity to learn insights from seniors who have experiences spanning many decades, while further developing their own potential to be sensitive and socially-conscious leaders. At the same time, as their elder partners begin to see how meaningful, interesting, and applicable their thoughts and reflections can be to a young person, they begin to realize that their lives really have mattered. As one college junior enthusiastically explained, "Being able to take a peek at what someone with many years of living has experienced and learning what is important to them is precious." Similarly, a retired college professor shared happily, "These are the most meaningful questions that anyone has ever asked me." The benefits of partnering a student interviewer with an older resident in order to better shape the latter's legacy for his/her loved ones are evident for both age groups.

Of course, the program's success and benefits depend on the training the students receive. Effective training begins with the creation of good partnerships: selecting students who are responsible, sociable, and self-identified "good writers" and then pairing them with residents who will enjoy working with students, and who have little to no long-term memory loss. Conducting a brief screening interview with all potential student participants helps identify those who most display maturity and leadership. Our experience has taught us that these qualities – rather than chronological age – are more reliable criteria for selecting appropriate student applicants. In addition, as we have noted elsewhere, increasing the number of participants does not necessarily make it a better program.[9] Although *Lessons of a Lifetime* was created with a research component in mind – with informed-consent forms to be signed by all participants – our suggestion is that all participants sign these forms, whether or not research will be taking place (parental signatures are also suggested for students under 18). This precaution promises strict confidentiality to the senior participants who are sharing personal and intimate knowledge about themselves. It also reminds the students that what they are hearing and recording must remain accessible only to staff involved with the project itself. Indeed, potential problems can be avoided when this explanation is part of a thorough and honest description of the ethical will interview process given to student trainees.[10]

Because of the nature of ethical wills and what they convey, and how an interviewee might respond to memories of certain life-episodes recalled, it is important that all interviewers have a working knowledge of the psychological and psychotherapeutic issues of concern to older

9   We found that a small group of 10 to 15 bright student volunteers suffices, and a larger group might be unwieldy and difficult to coordinate. Cf. our article "Sharing Wisdom and Building Community: The Ethical Will Project" in the February 2007 issue of *Long-Term Living*. (Search for our names at www.ltlmagazine.com.)

10   Before the program began, our facility's Institutional Review Board (IRB – which reviews research projects in order to protect residents who are the subjects of research conducted in our facility) gave formal approval for the program – including the informed consent forms – in order to formally assure everyone involved that the resident participants in the program would be treated with the utmost care and respect. One of the authors of this chapter (Hedy Peyser) is chairperson of the IRB, and recused herself for purposes of evaluating Lessons of a Lifetime™.

adults (i.e. dealing with loss, personal sense of meaning and purpose) and know how to respond to these appropriately. That is, interviewers need to recognize words and body language that signal a participant's distress, while also recognizing that it is not their responsibility, nor do they have the expertise, to treat or provide care for the participant. Among those who do have the expertise is the pastoral care provider. Although often intersecting with social workers, pastoral caregivers, as *de facto* representatives of God, can and are expected to help residents address questions of Ultimate Meaning. Helping residents to feel God's presence as they address these "big picture" questions, pastoral caregivers provide the "spiritual scaffolding" for residents as they construct their responses through the writing of an ethical will.[11]

Regarding the training session's length and breadth, certainly a more comprehensive training is always preferable to a less rigorous alternative. However, experience has taught us that, in addition to attending our facility's regular volunteer orientation, a two-hour training session specifically focused on ethical will interviewing is sufficient to ensure successful interviews and a positive experience for all participants.

Training The "Scribes"

The training that a student undergoes in order to be an effective *Lessons of A Lifetime* interviewer "scribe" consists of two parts. The first is a one-hour lecture focusing on the accurate and effective transcription of notes into the documents themselves, while the second is a one-hour practicum on gaining "hands-on" experience. The lecture's main objective is to familiarize students with the three major principles on which effective ethical will interviewing rests: neutrality, clarity, and reassurance.

The first principle, neutrality, is arguably the most important skill for the interviewer to develop. It is axiomatic that interviewers remain "non-judgmental" during the interview; they must be ever-mindful that they are not there to evaluate what the residents are sharing, but only to record what is being said as accurately as possible. This is particularly important when responses are being recorded with pen and paper, rather

---

11   For more on the difference between the respective roles of the social worker and chaplain, cf. Cary Kozberg's explanation of the chaplain's "priestly" role in his chapter "You Shall Be Holy: the Roles of the Chaplain in Senior Residential Care Settings".

than with a tape recorder, video camera, or an audio/visual computer program.[12] Unlike an interview that is recorded with audio/visual technology in which a person's body language, facial expression and tone of voice can be seen and heard, an interview in which the responses are recorded by hand must be such that the words of the interviewee speak for themselves, and not be skewed by the manner in which the interview is conducted.

For this reason, it is most important that student interviewers are careful not to communicate any bias through their own body language, facial expressions, or even in the way a particular comment is written down. Novice interviewers need to understand not only the necessity of refraining from making verbal judgments, but also how non-verbal cues can themselves communicate a judgmental response. For example, if an interviewer is visibly uncomfortable with a particular comment made by his/her interviewee, the interviewee may not be as forthcoming during the rest of interview. Such a response would not only indicate a disrespect for the interviewee's genuine feelings (which are an authentic part of what he/she is leaving), but also compromise the authenticity of the ethical will itself.

Another aspect of effective interviewing that is stressed during training is insuring clarity and keeping the interviewee focused. When relating emotional experiences, interviewees may confuse topics and/or the chronology of events. When this happens, the interviewer needs to ask gentle and respectful probing questions so that the interviewee's responses will be clear and easily understandable. In addition, as the interview is concluding, the interviewer should return to the central question "what have your life's experiences taught you?"[13] Ideally ethical wills should be written in the first person, in order to give them a warmer, more personal tone for the benefit of those to whom they are ultimately intended. Again, unlike oral histories, ethical wills are not just an objective reporting of past life events, but personal expressions of the major lessons learned from those events, and offered with the intention of providing practical life-wisdom to future generations.

It is also incumbent on the interviewer to understand the

---

12   This is done largely for simplicity's sake and to reduce costs. However, all interviewers are required to review the ethical will with the senior to ensure accuracy and correct any possible mistakes.

13   "A Volunteer's Guide to Recording Oral Histories and Ethical Wills©".

importance of reassuring and affirming the older interviewee as he/she responds to each question. Engaged students are usually very receptive to learning active listening skills and quickly come to recognize the importance of empathy when working with others. In this context these skills include:

- Acknowledging what the interviewee has communicated, both verbally and non-verbally.
- Summarizing what the interviewee has said to demonstrate attentiveness and ensure that the information is accurate.
- Asking probing questions to better understand what the interviewee means.
- Verbally affirming the interviewee's emotions in order to show empathy.
- Remaining quiet at key moments to allow time for thought and personal reflection.
- Being mindful of the interviewee's body language as well as one's own body language.
- Reassuring the interviewee that his/her responses are not being evaluated or judged and will remain strictly confidential.[14]

An ethical will is essentially a "love letter" to family and other loved ones – a gift that contains the lessons, insights and bits of practical advice gleaned from an entire life's experience. Understanding the importance of the above-mentioned skills helps students to be more attentive to the emotions of their senior participant-partners, and thereby help them create a gift that will be more precious.

Other logistical aspects of the training that will insure a smoother interview process also include:

- Understanding the voluntary (and open-ended) nature of both the interviewer's and interviewee's participation (i.e. either is free to withdraw at any time).
- Understanding the importance of maintaining strict confidentiality.
- Acquiring basic quick and accurate note-taking skills.
- Setting up the initial meeting between interviewer and

---

14   These and more can be found in *Lessons of a Lifetime*™, "A Volunteer's Guide to Recording Oral Histories and Ethical Wills©".

interviewee.

- Arranging for an appropriate interview venue to insure mutual privacy and comfort.
- Managing the interview time (at least two or three one-hour interviews are necessary).
- Reviewing interview notes with interviewees at the end of each session to ensure accuracy.
- Remaining in contact with the program administrators and/ or chaplain.
- Arranging for the production of the final draft of each ethical will.[15]

Although the particulars may vary based on the needs of the facility, it is important that administrators/supervisors of such a program discuss and clarify these details with their student trainees, making sufficient time for questions and discussion. (One way of sparking discussion and reviewing points that may still seem vague or unclear is to ask students "What are three things you would change about this presentation?") Of course, handouts of an outline and/or slides to a PowerPoint presentation are useful for the students' future reference.

With the conclusion of the didactical part of the training, the "hands-on" practicum can begin with students pairing up and beginning an exercise in which they record each other's ethical wills. One hour will not be sufficient for students to create complete, polished versions of what they would like to pass on. However, it will allow them to begin practicing their new skills and hopefully gain a stronger appreciation of how challenging and meaningful this exercise can be for both themselves and their residents.

During this exercise, it is important for the program's administrators to circulate among the trainees and address any questions that may arise. At the end of the practicum, some concluding remarks are appropriate, along with a request that students continue working with their partners to complete their respective ethical wills prior to starting work with the senior interviewees themselves. Once they have "recorded and been recorded" and have turned in their work (ideally within a few days of the training), they may be assigned to their respective residents to begin the work.

---

15   Cf. "The Use of Ethical Wills to Engage Future Jewish Leaders." *Religious Education*, Vol. 105:5, October – December 2010: pages 536 – 548.

Supervising And Celebrating "The Work"

As students begin to work with their interviewees, supervision of the program becomes relatively straightforward. Supervisors may decide to schedule regular weekly meetings between students and their senior interviewees in a set venue (this is preferable when the interviewees are residents of a senior care center). Alternatively, they may choose to let the pairs meet at time that is mutually convenient. Should an interviewer and interviewee choose the latter, it is recommended (with the safety of both parties in mind) that they *not* meet in a place that is completely secluded, but rather in a place where other staff are easily accessible – perhaps a quiet corner of a library or social hall.

Supervisors should make sure that the student interviewer reviews his/her notes after each session, and prepares them by the following day to ensure that the finished product will be as current and as accurate as possible. When supervising brand-new volunteers, it may be prudent to have them submit a brief summary about each session, checking with them to make sure that they feel adequately prepared and are not finding the process stressful or overly challenging. Similarly, supervisors should also check in with the residents being interviewed to make sure that they are finding the experience both enjoyable and fulfilling.

After a number of ethical wills have been created, it is suggested that the work of both the student interviewers and the senior interviewees be appropriately and formally recognized. Our facility holds an "Ethical Will Soirée" – a brief recognition ceremony followed by a dessert reception – to which friends and families of both the students and residents are invited. At the ceremony, students are recognized for their dedication and leadership, and residents are invited to present their ethical wills (printed and bound in a nice booklet) to their loved ones.

It is not surprising that this kind of ceremony can be quite emotional for all attending – students, residents, their families, the program administrators, and others who are invited. For the students, it affirms their substantive contribution to the lives of the older adults with whom they have become intimately acquainted. For the residents, it affords them the opportunity to feel that they have attained "a bit of immortality" by passing their wisdom on to the next generation. And for those who administer and supervise the program, it can deepen the sense of gratification that comes from knowing how much such a program edifies and enriches the lives of those for whom they care.

One of our fondest memories to date is something that happened at one of these soirees:

Frances was a 99-year-old resident and our oldest participant in the Lessons of a Lifetime *program. Although she enjoyed a very close relationship with her mother throughout her life, Frances's daughter was amazed at what her mother shared in her ethical will during the ceremony. "I never knew this about my mother," she noted excitedly. Moreover, Frances made an indelible impression on the student volunteer who had worked with her. After the project finished and their formal sessions concluded, their discussions about life still continued, and their relationship deepened. Frances died a few weeks before her 100th birthday. At her request, her ethical will was read at her funeral.*

From what we have experienced and learned in creating *Lessons of a Lifetime*, we believe that ethical wills can be an important part of the repertoire of chaplains, pastoral caregivers and other professionals who want to help nurture the spiritual lives of older adults. Moreover, when youths are engaged and trained to help seniors create them, ethical wills can serve as a unique way of breaking through the attitudes and prejudices that often encumber intergenerational dialogue. By enabling students and seniors to learn about each other as they work towards a common goal, they can impart a sense of meaning and purpose for both those at the beginning of their lives and those who are nearing the end of theirs. As a younger cohort helps an older cohort to transmit its wisdom to future generations, both can experience a taste of timelessness in the wisdom they share.

Chapter 19

A Picture's Worth 1000 Souls: Partnering Creative Arts Therapy And Jewish Spiritual Care

Deborah Ann Del Signore, M.A.A.T., ATR-BC

Although not Jewish, I have worked as an art therapist in a Jewish organization serving predominately Jewish elders in a senior residential care center for over a decade. Over the years I have worn many hats (sometimes simultaneously) including art therapist practitioner, manager of the facility's Creative Arts Therapies department, director of its Alzheimer's special care community and, most recently, manager of Life Enrichment Services. I have worked directly with residents and have been responsible for overseeing large programming projects. These experiences have afforded me many opportunities to witness the importance of spirituality for specific residents and for the senior residential community at large. As I have assisted residents explore the impact of Jewish traditions and culture on their lives, and watched how they have provided times to celebrate on Sabbaths and holidays, and times for solace and reflection when life is ending, I have seen how the presence of "creative arts therapies" can enhance, or at least "hold" the spiritual significance of these moments and thereby enhance their sanctity.

I work for CJE SeniorLife in Chicago, a comprehensive network of housing, healthcare, community services, education and applied research. Since 1972 it has enhanced the lives of older adults and their families throughout metropolitan Chicago. CJE Senior Life serves over 18,000 people each year.[1] Their skilled nursing facility is Lieberman

---

1   For more about CJE, cf. Susan Buchbinder's chapter "Cultural Competency in a Jewish-sponsored Senior Residential Care Setting".

Center for Health and Rehabilitation, located in Skokie, which is where I have spent the last decade of my professional career. Serving as many as 240 individuals on any given day, Lieberman offers various levels of care: skilled nursing, dementia care, short-term rehabilitation and end-of-life care. Some people call Lieberman their home; others come for short-term rehabilitation services and return home after their stay.

Today there are a variety of living options for older adults. Those who become residents of long-term care facilities like Lieberman tend to be the oldest of the old, the frailest of the frail. Yet, despite their age and frailty, many of these individuals still possess tremendous spiritual strength, and thus we must be careful not to assume they come to nursing homes simply to die. Indeed, it has been my privilege to watch many older, frail individuals rediscover themselves and in some instances reinvent themselves at this stage of their lives. (Readers are encouraged to read the mission statement of the department at the end of this chapter.)

By way of introduction, I want to briefly discuss some highlights of the movement toward "culture change" in senior residential care that is currently taking place in this country. It is a movement in which Lieberman is very much at the forefront – a movement which advocates the kind of change in which both pastoral care and creative arts therapies can and should play leading roles.

One of the desired outcomes of the culture change movement is to restore the focus on basic residents' rights that was inadvertently pushed into the background, over the last half-century or so, as older adults became "institutionalized". The traditional nursing home usually operates according to a "medical" model where sterile, regimented environments are considered to be most appropriate for the kind of care given. With less attention paid to resident rights, there has been an accompanying loss of focus on the person being cared for.

The culture change movement promotes the rights of individual residents to have a say in their care. It encourages facilities to help them to voice their opinions and keep everyday life tasks in a close locus of control: to be able to choose what they eat, when they eat, when they go to bed and when they wake up. In a word, it promotes the preservation of the same rights for nursing home residents that those who live independently enjoy, rights that many current residents also probably took for granted before becoming long-term care residents.[2]

---

2   For more on the "cultural change" movement in senior residential

At Lieberman, our belief is that the creation of relationships – between staff and residents, residents and residents, families and residents, families and staff – is of paramount importance to the health and quality of the culture we want to nurture for older adults in senior residential care settings. The creative arts therapies and a facility's religious/spiritual program both instill a sense of being part of something larger than oneself. Indeed, religion and the arts have repaired broken cultures of the past and influenced the development of new cultures throughout human history. What follows are examples of how our Creative Arts Therapy program[3] has elicited and supported the nurturing of the spiritual lives of our residents, and how we have partnered with those responsible for creating a vibrant and meaningful religious atmosphere – namely, our rabbi.

Jewish People And The Arts

A personal note: I have always been impressed with the importance of art in Jewish tradition and its appreciation among Jewish people.[4] When I first came to work at Lieberman, I immediately noticed the large number of original artworks – many with Jewish themes – that hung throughout the building. There was a wonderful collection of unique and, in some instances, very valuable pieces of art everywhere. The entire collection was the result of a committed cadre of very generous individuals who donated the pieces to the home. Working in such an environment, I knew that, as an art therapist, I would be supported in bringing opportunities for creative expression to the residents.

A key teaching related to the practice of Judaism is the concept

---

care, readers are encouraged to learn about the work of the Pioneer Network. (www.pioneernetwork.net)

3   It should be noted that the program referred to in this chapter is a creative arts *therapy* program, not merely a creative arts program. It is staffed exclusively by Master's-level professionals who are clinically trained to utilize "arts modalities and creative processes during intentional interventions in therapeutic, rehabilitative, community, or educational settings to foster health, communication and expression" in order to "promote the integration of physical, emotional, cognitive and social functioning; enhance self awareness, and facilitate change." (from NCCATA website)

4   Some time ago National Public Radio ran a story that members of the Jewish community give more money to the arts than any other religious cohort in the world. This did not surprise me and I have never forgotten it.

of *hiddur mitzvah* – making the commandment beautiful. What this means is that whenever someone is performing a specific religious duty, he/she should try to do so in a way that makes the experience more beautiful and aesthetically pleasing. So, for example, a Passover Seder plate should not be just a "plain" plate, but rather one that is specially decorated or artistically created for the Seder ceremony. In addition, the way that the ritual foods are placed on the Seder plate should also be intentional, with aesthetics as a main consideration.

One of the hallmarks of Jewish tradition is that it is filled with lots of rituals. Some of these occur daily or weekly, some annually and others only during certain rites of passage. As with the Seder plate used at Passover, many of these are performed with specific items associated, and in the spirit of *hiddur mitzvah*, many of these items are created as beautiful *objects d'art* in and of themselves. These items include but are not limited to:

- *menorahs* (candelabrums used for Hanukah)[5]
- *mezuzahs* (objects affixed to the doorposts with the verses from Deuteronomy 6:4 placed inside)
- Sabbath candlesticks and covers for *challah* (the special bread eaten on the Sabbath)
- hand washing cups, used before sitting down to a meal
- hand-fashioned pointers (*yad* – a tool in the shape of pointing finger used to read the Torah scroll)
- *kippot* (skullcaps)
- *tallitot* (prayer shawls)

Not only do these objects resonate aesthetically with residents, they often strike a powerful spiritual chord as well. I have worked with people who have found significant meaning and comfort in re-creating ritual objects from their past, or in making new ones for use in the present. Both keep them connected to the religious tradition that came before them – and will continue after they are gone. The effect of this blending of the arts and religious tradition on individuals was

---

5   Menorahs from the 19th and 20th centuries can be very ornate and elaborate (often commissioned by wealthy individuals), or very simple (reflecting the modest circumstances of poor *shtetl* life in Eastern Europe). However, although the latter are often modest, they are invariably quite beautiful.

powerfully illustrated by one woman I will call Miriam.

A short-term rehab resident, Miriam was passing the art studio one day and noticed that we did not have a *mezuzah* on the door, and decided then and there to make one for us. Coming to the studio every day after her physical therapy session, she sculpted, painted and fired her ceramic mezuzah. Then, with the assistance of the rabbi, she obtained the appropriate religious script to place inside the *mezuzah* and hung the *mezuzah* on the door of the studio. Although brief and mostly focused on her physical rehabilitation, Miriam's stay at Lieberman was enriched by her commitment to Jewish tradition and art making. Her spirit as well as her body became stronger as she gained a renewed purpose and meaning (a major goal of culture change). And when she returned for other stays at Lieberman, she always came to the studio to take a peek at *her mezuzah*. Working with Miriam, I saw again how art is so naturally woven into the fabric of Jewish life, and how experiences like this can influence Jewish older adults to access the arts as a vehicle for emotional and spiritual healing and support.

Arts, Meaning, And God

As a person ages and the productive days of adulthood give way to more time spent reviewing one's life, there tends to be a new search for meaning and the asking of existential questions: *Why am I here? What is/was my purpose?* Of course, the answers to these questions are never objective but subjective, and in their search people may turn to therapy and/or religion. In some forms of therapy with older adults the concept of a "God" or a Higher Power is often intrinsic to a person's search for meaning – which itself is affirmed by several theories of human development as being necessary in later life.

For example, I once worked with a woman who explored the meaning of God often through the imagery she created in her painting, as well as in our discussions together. She reflected on the challenges she faced in her life, specifically her lifelong struggle with bi-polar disorder (which caused several hospitalizations during her nine decades) and the premature death of her husband and adult child. She was trying to make sense of her life and come to a comfortable resolution of why she was asked to carry these burdens. She decided to turn to God, "in His glory and mystery". One of the images she painted was of an autumn tree on a grassy knoll under the brilliant light of a blue sky. She was exploring the concept of "the god within" and how it can be very much entwined with the self. She explained:

> *I think that painting has done a lot for me. I would want people to get a feeling of color when they look at my painting. This painting gives off the feeling of being one with nature. I think that you get a feeling that you are with G-d (sic). I tried to capture the colors of the sky, the ground and a storm might be coming in. I really like the sky. I think that colors are the things that an artist should get at, as well as the pathos and the happiness of the person that is making it. I think people have to paint with emotion. If they have no emotion how can they paint? I put down what I feel in my heart.*

Some believe, as do I, that all of our expressions are a direct portrait of our Self at any given moment in time. This woman was at the stage of development in which her reflections supported the notion that the sense of Self and the sense of God can be experienced as almost indistinguishable from one another.

Nature was a common motif in this woman's art. She also frequently juxtaposed polarities in her work. For example, she might express a fretful anticipation of a storm with a calm appreciation of the beauty of a landscape. One memorable example of her juxtaposing polarities was one particular image in which she expressed both praise and fear of God. She depicted a woman being engulfed by beautiful, yet turbulent waters caused by an impending storm …

> *The turbulence of Nature's own art … the miracle of what "G-d" performs … Do we dare face the fury of Mother Nature?*

This is just one example of an art-based response to some of life's "ultimate questions", which may include various existential quandaries and/or conversations with God. All are quests to find meaning and purpose in a life that is drawing to a close. Unfortunately, in traditional senior care settings there has been little support offered to residents to help them explore and process these developmentally necessary thoughts and feelings. Yet, from what the few examples offered above show, such support can obviously make a huge difference in a resident's psychological, emotional and spiritual well-being. For this reason, it seems obvious that similar programs are called for in whatever group settings older adults reside. Indeed, these examples also show that the big questions about life do not have to be explored exclusively within the "religious and spiritual" realm. On the contrary, the methods and approaches offered by the creative arts – specifically image-making and creative writing – present a unique compliment to more "traditional" religious and spiritual approaches: they offer a vehicle by which people can continue their individual searches for meaning in ways that are unique and transformative.

Art, Religion And Identity

As an arts therapist, I understand my role as one of assisting clients to find the best, most accessible creative medium for them, and then provide a safe and supportive environment for self-expression to occur. I tend not to give directives when working in groups or with individual clients; I believe we can find the content of our art within ourselves, and that the content chosen is what matters most to us at any given moment. Following the writings of the late gerontologist Robert Butler, an arts room should be a place that encourages the natural tendency of individuals to review their lives as they get older, for the purposes of resolving life issues. In my work, I have seen many people do this, using Jewish culture as a guide and set of reference points. This happens in many ways.

Some re-image stories from the Torah that they have heard throughout their lives. For instance, one woman fashioned a very intricate clay sculpture of Mount Sinai with a bearded Moses carrying the tablets of the Ten Commandments down the mountain. A few people have drawn or sculpted a burning bush. Noah's Ark, with pairs of every animal she could think of, was one woman's project for many months. Paintings of the parting of the Red Sea have also been popular.

Sometimes the memories and events that residents explore are more specific and more personal. One woman who was unable to attend her grandson's wedding sculpted a multi-media bride and groom standing under the *chuppah* (wedding canopy).

Exploring Jewish Identity Through Film

Five years ago we started a film program, called *Inner Views*. Its purpose is to create 30-minute interview-based documentaries about the residents living at Lieberman. The recorded resident interviews are viewed by all direct care staff, so that they can learn more about the lives of individual residents. In this way relationships between caregivers and residents will improve (as will care practices) and the sense of community in the nursing home will be strengthened.

To be sure, the project has proven to be most dynamic and has several positive effects that are beyond the purview of this chapter. However, one relevant effect has shown how creating such documentary films can serve as an outlet for residents expressing their Jewish identity. During these interviews, many participants discuss honestly and authentically what it has meant to them to be Jewish, or how being Jewish affected their lives. In one film, a resident shared his story about being a young Jewish man during World War II. Although he really wanted serve in the army, he was rejected due to his weight and had to work in a factory making bullets. Wanting to do his part back home so that soldiers serving "in the wilderness" would have all that they needed to protect themselves, he made sure the machines worked at full capacity. In return for his hard work, his fellow workers taunted him for being Jewish. Unbeknownst to him, they would place "rejection slips" on his back that indicated that he was Jewish, and therefore a "reject". During the making of the film, this gentleman told the interviewer that he was so saddened and upset by this taunting, that he "actually cried". But the story had a happier ending: eventually he was accepted into the army after quitting the job at the factory and spoke about how proud he was to finally be able to "fight the fight".

In another film, a survivor of the Holocaust shared her entire story of what happened to her during that terrible time, parts of which she had never shared with her family. Because of this program, she was able to tell her story of how as a teenager she lived alone in the woods for months, having to pretend to be someone she was not because she "was afraid to say (she) was Jewish". Although this woman passed away very soon after her story was filmed and screened, the sorrow felt at her passing was mitigated by the joy that she had finally been able to share her terrible ordeal with others, in a safe and nurturing environment.

Jewish Identity And Practice For Persons With Dementia

As arts therapists we believe that, although cognitive capacities may weaken or be lost, the essence of a person is always present. Thus, even though cognitive losses may inhibit effective self expression, our responsibility as arts therapists is to provide guidance and opportunities that foster self-expression, and thus keep individuals connected to their religious and cultural heritage. In my work over the years with Jewish residents, I have found that tapping into a person's Jewish identity is a very effective way to help that person express him/herself, even when he/she is living with severe dementia, as the following examples attest.

When an expressive therapist (an arts therapist who incorporates a variety of art modalities into their practice) visited our memory care community, he was able to visibly engage Jewish members of that community by having them sit around a Passover table and reenact relationships with significant loved ones who were no longer alive. During the exercise, they were also able to recall and access the details of the Passover Seder meal and rituals which made the program even richer and more edifying for them.

Creating worship experiences that have been adapted to their particular situations is another important way of keeping Jewish individuals with dementia connected to their religious and cultural heritage.

For the past few years our music therapist has partnered with a volunteer (the wife of a local rabbi) to conduct High Holiday services specifically for persons living with moderate to severe dementia. With this population, a standard worship service is usually too long and/or too complicated to follow. With her knowledge of dementia and how to engage those with significant cognitive impairment, the music therapist created a worship experience which enables this population to be active worshipping participants during these most sacred days of the year. The adapted services are held in a residential part of the home with a more intimate ambience, and are much shorter in length (45 minutes as opposed to the two-plus hours in the synagogue).

Music is an extremely important part of this experience because it taps effortlessly into the needs and strengths of persons living with dementia. During these adapted High Holiday services, prayers recited daily are chanted, and familiar songs specific to the traditional High Holiday liturgy are also added to help those present better identify with both the experience and the season, while also feeling successful while participating. Of course, active participation is encouraged and often opportunities for reminiscing are incorporated to help those present feel more successful and "connected".

Another (favorite) example of "connecting": A few years ago we had a drama therapist visit the residents of our Alzheimer's Special Care Community on a regular basis. I'll never forget walking past his group one day and watching as a woman, who was for all intents and purposes non-verbal and confined to a wheelchair, stood up, held an imaginary wine glass and exclaimed "*L'chaim!*"[6]

End Of Life

During my time here at Lieberman, some of the most spiritual moments I have experienced have occurred when life is ending. I have sat with people who were dying, as their families held hands and, with the help of a music therapist, sing songs as their loved one took his/her last breath. I have also seen that just as individuals turn to religion toward the end of life, sometimes they are also supported and nurtured in this last life passage by remaining creative and making art. During the last months and days, there is often a clear transformation, evidenced by their changed facial expressions, which is humbling to witness.

I remember one particular resident who was a woman coping with a diagnosis of terminal cancer. In the last three months of her life I assisted her in an image and poetry-making life review that ranged from exploring her relationship with her beloved dog and members of her family to her travels around the United States in an RV with her husband. This was an emotionally rich time in her life, filled with tears and laughter. Under her direction we made a portfolio of her work, which she requested to be given to her son upon her death. As she grew weaker during her last few weeks she would leave her bed only to come to the art therapy group twice a week. The day before she died she turned to her son and said, "If this is D-E-A-T-H, then there is nothing to be afraid of." I cannot help but believe that the reason she had come to accept her impending death was largely due to the creative life review upon which she had embarked in her final months.

Opportunities To Collaborate

Weaving Jewish spiritual care together with the creative arts makes direct collaboration with the rabbi/chaplain indispensable. This partnership between the members of Creative Arts Therapy department and the rabbi/chaplain here at Lieberman has taken many forms over the years. But in all of its forms, it is a partnership that I have always valued.

---

6   The traditional Jewish toast. *L'chaim!* means "to life!". For more on responding to the needs of Jewish individuals with dementia, cf. Ellen Cahn's chapter "Judaism and Dementia".

Since both departments respond to the reality of death regularly, one area for significant and ongoing collaboration has been around the creation of a ritual of remembrance to honor deceased residents. This includes a memorial service which is conducted by the rabbi, along with our transforming the synagogue into a gallery in which the deceased resident's artwork is shown. This allows family and loved ones to grieve their loss in a traditional manner, but at the same time celebrate the life and creative energy of the person being remembered.

Another unique example of our collaborative efforts was the creation of a weekly group combining arts therapy and pastoral care that the rabbi and I would facilitate together. I will admit that perhaps my initial enthusiasm was a bit "selfish." Not only was this a great way to address issues of religion and spirituality that clients often bring to our work together, but it was also a wonderful opportunity for me to increase my limited knowledge of Judaism. And the fact that the rabbi played the guitar made this combination of the arts and religion all the more fitting!

Our plan was to focus on some well known selections from the Book of Psalms through group discussion and art-making. We began each session with music to set the mood, which led into the reading of the particular psalm for that week. The reading was followed by a group discussion which dissected certain verses within the psalm. The last part of the experience was to express, through drawing, any personal responses – thoughts or feelings – that the verses and/or discussion elicited.

The group was both exciting and unique in purpose, content and makeup, since many of the people who decided to join us were not the "regulars" in the studio. Instead, they were predominately those who participated in the religious life offerings at Lieberman, and reflecting on their religious and spiritual "selves" through drawing was a new experience for all of them. Expecting some of them to be resistant to art making, I was pleasantly surprised when consistently everyone participated fully in all of the parts of the group experience.

This consistency on the part of the participants may have been a function of the consistency of each session. The reading of the psalm was followed by a simple question "What does this mean?" to elicit cognitive responses. The drawings, on the other hand, focused on responses that were more affective, by helping to apply the determined meaning of the psalm to personal experiences and reflection. Indeed, the program's worth was seen not only in *who* participated, but also in their responses: many expressed both astonishment and gratitude at being able not only to connect with a part of their Jewish heritage heretofore unknown, but also experiencing it in ways that were gratifying and healing.

Religious Life, Creative Arts Therapies, And Building Community

In our effort to strengthen a sense of community among those who live and work at Lieberman, our Creative Arts Therapy team has put together several arts-based projects, with some of these projects having a Jewish religious component to them. They may be as simple as the spontaneous singing of holiday songs during Passover or Hanukah, (perhaps with a particular resident as the leader), contributing a resident's artwork for CJE's Rosh Hashanah card, or facilitating a resident "band" to play musical instruments during weekly religious services. Others involve a bit more planning and effort – such as our project in which older adult artists from among CJE's clients explored what it meant to be Jewish through a collection of murals that were displayed in a downtown Chicago gallery.

Some of our art and religious-based community building projects take place over longer periods of time which create opportunities for several gatherings. Sometimes they are "collective works" in which several hands (and hearts) contribute to the same image. Our *Tree of Life Project* was just such a project, and has proven to be a wonderful example of how the arts can be used within a senior residential care setting to create a stronger sense of community through the exploration of spiritually significant topics.

The Tree of Life Community Building Project was a 12-month, multi-sensory, interdisciplinary exploration of the "tree of life", a familiar Jewish theme. The overall design was created by our Creative Arts Therapy team, while the small group experiences were facilitated by members of the Life Enrichment Services team. The creative arts therapists worked with a leadership group of residents who made decisions about the final art piece and the general progress of the program at large. Discussions about the spiritual and religious significance of this theme in Jewish culture and teachings were led by our rabbi. The project culminated in a large-scale artwork for our community, a multi-media work on canvas, 9 feet tall x 6.5 feet wide.

We divided the year-long project into several metaphorically rich

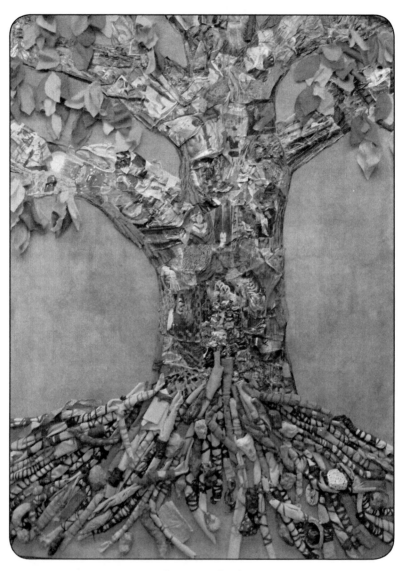

The Tree of Life

phases based on the parts of the tree: *Seeds: Wishes for the Future; Roots: Personal Traditions; Trunk: Strength; Leaves: The Circle of Life*. Each phase incorporated story, music, ritual, and art-making and was thoughtfully designed and executed to engage participants in the Tree of Life topic, with its connections to nature/natural processes, the human life cycle/ seasons of life, spirituality/Judaism, and our human experience of time (past, present, and future). Over 120 participants had the opportunity to create a multi-media art piece to be later incorporated into the overall Tree of Life image on canvas.

To initiate each phase of our Tree of Life project, the rabbi led the CJE community in exploring Jewish and spiritual issues by sharing scholarly knowledge and traditional wisdom to deepen the participants' spiritual connection to the Tree of Life. Throughout the different phases, he connected the themes explored in small groups to Jewish history, tradition, custom, and story. The residents listened and added their own thoughts in response to his description of the various trees in the Garden of Eden and to the Talmudic tale of the olive tree planted in the present to benefit future generations. Together, the rabbi and the participants shared thoughts about the Jewish life cycle and the life of a tree – how each part of a tree is much like a part of our self. Expanding this theme, the rabbi compared each resident's individual importance and contribution to the world to that of the Tree of Life.

The final product was unveiled in a final celebration to a packed room of community members, staff, family and volunteers just prior to the Jewish High Holidays. The Tree of Life project was a tremendous success in bringing the community together by searching out the religious and spiritual meanings of "the circle of life" through the arts. Today the "Tree" hangs proudly in our synagogue and continues to be a source of inspiration, especially during Shabbat and holiday celebrations.

Conclusion

This chapter contains examples of programs that are possible and necessary if the culture of long-term care for older adults is to be transformed into something that affirms the lives and dignity of its residents. I truly believe that the disciplines of creative arts therapies and religious life/spiritual care can be keys in making this much needed change happen. In our own unique ways we can provide a vehicle for a comfortable passage through the last stages of life – a time when existential questions – which sometimes have no answer – come to the forefront and invite inner reflection. In this way, we can also offer opportunities to individuals to carefully and meaningfully explore their beliefs about this life and perhaps the next. Collaboratively, our two disciplines can promote the creation and maintenance of relationships among all those who live in, work at, or visit the communities we serve. I hope our experience will inspire other creative arts therapists and chaplains to come together to support and enrich the emotional, social and spiritual well-being of Jewish elders living in similar settings, today and tomorrow.

Vision Statement Of CJE Senior Life's Creative Arts Therapies Department At The Lieberman Facility

Creative Arts Therapy at CJE Senior Life promotes personal growth and change by using art forms and clinical methods for individual and group therapy in an innovative, collaborative environment, executed cohesively across the continuum of care. We engage our clients through practices that integrate mind-body-spirit, build community and invite them toward self-discovery, awareness, and healing. As leaders in our field, we strive to be a best-practice, research-based discipline that empowers our clients, fosters well-being and independence, and sets the standard for creativity and innovation in eldercare. We will be recognized as the premier model for providing Creative Arts Therapy for older adults in metropolitan Chicago and beyond.

Creative Arts Therapy at Lieberman Center for Health and Rehabilitation uses the arts therapeutically to actively engage community members and improve quality of life through personalized interventions based on individual goals.

We provide three main areas of service: Clinical, Wellness and Community Building through the Arts.

Clinical services are provided to individuals with special psychological and/or physical needs and are referral driven. Both group and individual sessions are designed to meet these needs.

Wellness experiences are open to the general Lieberman Community and provide meaningful arts-based opportunities for self-expression, self-exploration and socialization.

Community Building through the Arts programming facilitates connections and creates a stronger sense of belonging among Lieberman community members by coming together and using the arts to work toward a shared goal.

Resources To Find A Creative Arts Therapist

American Art Therapy Association: www.arttherapy.org
American Music Therapy Association: www.musictherapy.org
American Dance / Movement Therapy Association: www.adta.org
National Association for Drama Therapy: www.nadt.org

Chapter 20

Playing Dreidel: A Unique "Spin" On Combining Jewish Holidays And Rehabilitative Therapies

Kate Brown

Working as a rehabilitation director in a skilled nursing environment presents challenges unique to the position: managing quality care, scheduling clients, and ensuring proper staffing patterns are among the tasks a rehab director is charged with throughout the work week. When I was hired to supervise the therapy department of a Jewish senior residential center, I imagined that the cultural aspects of the facility would add yet another layer of challenges to my position. I was certainly correct, and navigating those challenges in many ways defined my tenure as the manager there. What I did not realize prior to my first day was that embracing those challenges, and working within them, would create some of the most memorable treatment sessions I have observed as a professional in the field.

My company, Genesis Rehab Services (GRS) provides physical, occupational and speech therapies to clients with various rehabilitation needs. Physical therapy is primarily concerned with improving a person's functional mobility. PT focuses on such tasks as walking, moving in a wheelchair, prosthesis fitting, and lower body splinting. Occupational therapy addresses the tasks of every day living. OT works with clients on the tasks of grooming, dressing, bathing, and home management. Speech therapy focuses on communication skills as well as on the improvement of chewing and swallowing.

One of the sites with which GRS contracts to manage its therapy delivery is Wexner Heritage Village in Columbus, Ohio. In my capacity as site supervisor, I managed all three therapy disciplines within the center. During my time as manager, GRS issued a mandate to its rehab directors to increase the amount of time clients were treated in groups because of the benefits to be gained when patients are grouped together for rehab activities. For the clinician, grouping clients fosters better time management. For the client, it allows opportunities to see others working on similar goals and a chance to communicate about successes and frustrations. Within an institutional environment, it can also give a respite from the all-too-frequent feelings of isolation that is often experienced in a health care environment by creating a space for socialization.

For these reasons, our rehab team enthusiastically "bought into" the idea. However, translating the theoretical mandate into therapeutic practice was a bit more challenging. A natural planning structure for group therapy focuses on a theme. A theme keeps everyone engaged, patient and therapist alike. To be sure, when the clients are adults, themes need to be dignified and reflect their respective skill levels; themes that are perceived as "childish" are liable to detract from the therapeutic targets and thus need to be avoided. In order to follow our mandate, our team cycled through many ideas, and facilitated some great groups. But to keep up the interest of all concerned – clients and therapists alike – we were always looking for new ideas to meet our goals.

A significant weakness in our group curriculum was the inclusion of themes centered on holidays and holiday celebrations. Holidays are frequently incorporated into therapy groups in long-term care facilities, because all clients can relate to them, regardless of diagnosis. By sharing familiar experiences and memories through a theme like Christmas or Thanksgiving, clients naturally bond together. In addition, for many of our folks, holiday memories are joyful, and recalling them will often increase their participation for therapy tasks. But beyond these very significant reasons for selecting holidays as a therapy theme, there is also a subtler motivation. Happiness facilitates healing, and by tapping into a larger "consciousness of connection" consisting of family memories, seasonal events, and traditions, clients get some respite from a steady focus on their illnesses, by being reminded of *why* they want to be stronger and healthier.

But our team had an additional challenge: our particular senior residential center is under Jewish auspices; its mission is based on Jewish religious and cultural values. Consequently, we knew that we could not host the kind of "more familiar" therapeutic holiday-themed activities that might be offered at other centers, such as a Christmas tree-trimming group to improve balance or a Valentine-making group for fine finger skills. But what might we offer instead? The benefits of using holiday themes were too important to ignore. I decided to stop concentrating on what we could *not* do within the facility, and instead looked at the unique opportunities the Jewish culture afforded. I decided to use our challenges as tools for therapy planning. Perhaps we could not rely on familiar non-Jewish holiday concepts to motivate our clients, but we could accomplish the same goals *and* create an atmosphere of celebration by incorporating the holidays in the Jewish calendar into our agenda.

One afternoon, I approached one of our occupational therapists and asked for support in planning a group that would focus on the Jewish holiday of Shavuot, which commemorates the giving of the Ten Commandments. I asked the rabbi at our facility if it was acceptable that we celebrate the holiday within our therapy groups. He offered complete support and gave us some ideas as to what kinds of activities might be helpful to our patients. Implementing this program sounded so simple, and I asked myself: why hadn't the department been doing this kind of thing all along?

And yet, it felt "revolutionary." Although the center is a Jewish faith-based facility, it opens its doors to patients of all faiths. Thus, many of our clients and group participants are not Jewish and may know very little about the Jewish tradition. In addition, no therapy staff member is Jewish. As a team we were naturally concerned that our own ignorance would cause offensive missteps. We also wondered how clients would feel about celebrating holidays outside of their own faiths, and did not want our attempts at creative rehabilitation to be considered efforts to "convert our caseload" to Judaism. It was not at all apparent that we would be successful, but the program worked … and brilliantly.

One of the holiday customs associated with Shavuot is the eating of dairy foods. The reason is that milk is a symbol of nourishment and as milk nourishes the body, God's revelation nourishes the soul. With this in mind, we decided to celebrate with a favorite Shavuot delicacy – cheesecake and fruit. Food preparation naturally facilitates key target areas for occupational therapy, including organization for home management tasks, fine motor control, and sequencing. As part of the preparation, our therapists provided information about the holiday –

why it is observed, how it is celebrated – in written format to the group participants.

What we learned from the first group was that people wanted to learn about other Jewish holidays, and more about Jewish culture. In addition, we noted with particular interest that even if certain holidays are not from a client's own faith tradition, still the mere celebration of holidays in general helps remind participants of the goals toward which they are working. They are powerful reminders of home, family, and a normal and purposeful life. Realizing this made us want to continue.

The group that focused on Rosh Hashanah, the Jewish New Year, was one of our most successful groups. Completely conceptualized by one of our certified occupational therapy assistants, Yvonne Williams, this holiday program gave the therapists a joyful way to help participants improve a multitude of skills, including but not limited to, reaching, activity tolerance, fine motor skills, standing, sequencing, and planning. To help introduce the activity and set the right "spiritual" tone, the rabbi spoke to the patients about Rosh Hashanah's focus on change and personal improvement and sounded the *shofar* (ram's horn).

After learning about the holiday, the patients then created platters decorated with holiday symbols including stars of David, the *shofar*, and Hebrew sayings expressing themes of the holiday. Patients with appropriate safety awareness sliced apples and helped serve honey, traditionally eaten to celebrate the sweetness of the new year. In keeping with the theme of change and personal improvement, participants also reflected on what they wanted to accomplish in the coming year. After writing their thoughts on leaf-shaped paper, they were encouraged and assisted as needed to walk to a tree picture and paste their individual leaves on to the branches. These remained on display for the rest of the year.

Just as with Shavuot and Rosh Hashanah, Hanukah was likewise celebrated with clients of all faiths. During the Yuletide season, when many of us were making plans for Christmas Eve church services and buying stocking stuffers, focusing on an unfamiliar holiday perhaps should have felt foreign. But the opposite was true. In the spirit of the season, I felt the joy in our department multiply. I recall saying to one client, "I am spoiled working here. I get to celebrate double holidays!" She laughed and agreed. By this time, feeling more comfortable with incorporating Jewish holidays into our clinical practice, we all felt enriched by each season's celebrations.

In the spirit of the Hanukah holiday, the therapists indulged in a bit of seasonal fun, and allowed patients to "gamble" with beans as they played the traditional *dreidel* game. One particular client who was Jewish offered pointers to his small group and, spinning the *dreidel* with experienced flair, yelled, "Papa needs a new pair of shoes!" Not surprisingly, that got a hugely enthusiastic response from staff and other patients. But facilitating the *dreidel* game was not just a fun activity to celebrate the holiday. From a therapy perspective, it gave participants the opportunity to practice functional reaching, standing, fine motor skills, common math skills, and problem solving.

As is often the case when disparate ideas are brought together, the grafting of Jewish culture onto therapeutic rehabilitation inspired staff from both these disciplines to begin thinking about new and creative ways to better serve clients. One additional idea was a kosher cooking group, suggested to me by the facility's *mashgiach* (supervisor of kosher practices). She made suggestions about what foods might be prepared, and "kashered" (made ritually fit) all of the cooking implements by taking them to the *mikveh*.[1] Another idea came from one of our therapists, who, while doing some personal shopping, found a memory game in Hebrew and purchased it for the department. It was used successfully to help distract patients from the tedium that is often felt when they practice standing. In addition, Star of David sun catchers, crafted by some of our clients, decorated the rehab area's window, thus making it a brighter, more inviting, and more encouraging atmosphere.

Having been a part of this experiment, I can say without exaggeration that systematically weaving Jewish religious and cultural themes into the department's overall program changed the department. Not only was it a challenge, to learn the customs and traditions and their meanings, but it also significantly changed how we as a department normally operate. It made us come together to learn and grow not only as individuals, but also (and perhaps more importantly) as a team.

---

1   Editor's note: Biblical law states that certain people and objects that are ritually "pure" (*tahor*) may become ritually impure (*tamei*) for various reasons. A *mikveh* is a "ritual bath" used to help transform a person or object that is ritually impure to being ritually pure again. Immersion in a *mikveh* makes non-kosher cooking utensils kosher, and is also the last step in formal conversion to Judaism. In this way it is much like a baptismal pool. Religiously-observant Jewish women also immerse themselves in the *mikveh* after their menstrual cycles.

Moreover, it integrated us into the facility in a way previously not possible. Because we are not employed by the facility directly, but rather work for a company with which the facility contracts for therapy services, there is somewhat of a felt "separation" between us and the rest of the facility: we have always been "**in** the center," but have not necessarily been "**of** the center." By adopting parts of the center's core Jewish culture into our own mission and practices, we have facilitated a stronger and richer relationship between our clients and ourselves. The focus is now less about things like "contracts and reimbursement" and more about how can better co-operate to help the patients for whom we care.

There is one more important point to make. In the discipline of rehabilitation, we speak often about the "therapeutic use of self." The idea, credited to Anne Cronin Mosely, is that through rapport development, empathy, and honesty, therapists can achieve positive outcomes with our patients. There is a similar Jewish idea in the teachings of Hasidism called *yehidut*. *Yehidut* describes a transaction between a disciple (*hasid*) and his master (*rebbe*) during which the disciple learns from, and is helped by his master. In both of these helping phenomena, the encounter is understood to be greater than the participants themselves. This is because it is the *relationship* between them that matters; it is the mutual "give-and-take" that is therapeutic, fostering growth, and facilitating healing.

As this program proceeded we came to better appreciate the truth and wisdom behind this concept. Depending on the particular aspect of any given activity ("Jewish" or "rehabilitative"), there was a dynamic shift between who was "master" and who was "disciple". Thus, because "Judaism and Jewish traditions" was a topic unfamiliar to both the therapists and many of the clients, therapists and clients alike were "disciples" looking to the rabbi as "master" when he spoke on the religious meanings of the various holidays. By the same token, the rabbi and the clients found themselves in the role of "disciple" when it came to learning from the therapist ("master") about how playing the simple game of *dreidel* facilitates improving fine motor skills. To be sure, there is a certain vulnerability that is created when teacher/student roles are fluid in this way. But the vulnerability hopefully creates a mutual trust between "disciple" and "master" that in turn nurtures the empathy, honesty, and rapport development that are needed in the best therapeutic relationships.

By integrating Jewish traditions and customs into our therapy and by appreciating the parallels between the concept of *yehidut* and what makes for an effective therapeutic relationship, we were able to have meaningful and mutually beneficial relationships with our clients – who certainly experienced better outcomes as a result of the genuine passion we had for our newly learned activities. But perhaps more importantly, we also learned how to better use our "selves" as therapeutic tools to develop relationships not only with those who come to us for help, but with our colleagues as well. All people, regardless of what faith tradition they affirm, look to their holidays to "benchmark" their year. At their core, holidays are about people coming together. In our therapy work, we have come to appreciate that phenomenon with our clients and colleagues in new ways – for the betterment of us all.

Chapter 21
Being Thy Brother's Keeper: Ministry To People Of The Jewish Faith In A Christian Faith-Based Facility

Rev. Jim Jensen

Mrs. Shapiro[1] moved into our Assisted Living facility on a Friday afternoon. The chaplain knew from admission documents that she was Jewish, but he was not able to make an initial visit with her before leaving for the day. On Sunday morning, he was somewhat surprised to see her at the Christian worship service provided each week in the chapel, and felt a bit embarrassed about not having been able to inform her that this was a *Christian* worship service. On Monday, he visited her and apologized for not having informed her ahead of time that the worship service in the chapel was "Christian centered". She said, "No need to apologize. I can get something out of it!" Getting to know Mrs. Shapiro better, this author learned through subsequent conversations that she did indeed "get something out of it" which she could apply to her own life and faith.

Even as a Jew, Mrs. Shapiro had the capacity to see things in the Christian worship service that were quite meaningful to her own life and faith – something this author has also learned by attending the Jewish Sabbath and other holiday services that have been provided by the facility, with the help of local rabbis and laypersons.

To be sure, providing ministry to people of the Jewish faith in a Christian faith-based residential care facility – whose chaplain preaches and teaches the Christian faith – can present some unique challenges and opportunities. Jewish residents have specific spiritual and religious

---

1   Not her real name.

needs and expectations, but even in a Christian based facility – with adequate education, awareness and understanding on the part of the facility's chaplain and staff – these needs and expectations can be sensitively addressed.

However, what is of utmost priority is that all residents of a senior residential care community, regardless of their faith tradition, or lack of one, must be ministered to as individuals, as persons – with feelings and memories, with traditions and spiritual needs which have shaped them. Therefore, as every student chaplain learns, listening is **the** primary mode of ministry. Active listening and reflection are what allows the chaplain to discover who the person is, and what are his/her concerns, issues, needs, fears, and celebrations. It is through active listening and reflection that the chaplain is introduced to another's identity, spirituality and center of being.

When a resident of a senior residential care facility identifies himself or herself as "Jewish", there are some important things for which one must listen, and from which one must learn. Much can be gained in knowing what pastoral care issues need to be addressed by listening. As within American Christendom, there are many religious "streams" within the American Jewish community, and so Jewish residents may come from various traditions. Thus, a Christian chaplain working with Jewish residents should learn about these various streams and traditions within the Jewish faith, which of course can be achieved through both formal and informal inquiry and research.

Indeed, one significant and helpful truth that this author has come to learn is that, for the most part, there is no single Jewish position on any issue or belief. On the contrary, there is a wide variety of views regarding matters of belief, spirituality and religious life. Connection to Jewish history and the past and adhering to traditions that have been handed down from generation to generation are paramount, as is a strong sense of feeling connected to others in the Jewish community.

At a seminar presented at the 2008 Annual Conference of the Association of Professional Chaplains, Rabbi Fred M. Raskind, LPC-GA, shared some selective questions that non-Jewish chaplains can ask Jewish residents and clients in order to ascertain their religious and/or spiritual needs:

- Please share some of your religious practices.
- Did you grow up in an observant home?

- What dietary rules do you follow, such as avoiding *treif*, mixing milk and meat? Do you eat meat that is not kosher?
- If you had *Bar (m) / Bat (f) Mitzvah*, how do you remember it?
- With which group are you most comfortable: Orthodox, Conservative, Reform, or Reconstructionist? Why so?
- Do you identify more as a "cultural Jew"? Tell me more.
- Which holidays do you celebrate (*Rosh Hashanah, Yom Kippur, Succot, Hanukah, Purim, Passover, Shavuot*)? Which is your favorite?
- What were your grandparents like?
- Did / do you have relatives living nearby?
- How do you see yourself "Jewishly"? What makes you Jewish?
- Do you believe in an Ultimate Power?
- What is important for end-of-life rituals?
- Do you wish to be visited by a rabbi?

Once the chaplain has learned the answers to these and other questions that may seem important, he/she can sensitively begin to provide pastoral care to that individual.

One tradition observed by most Jews is to place a *mezuzah* on the outside door post of their home/apartment/room. The *mezuzah* contains a piece of parchment inscribed in Hebrew with verses from Deuteronomy 6: 4-9, the last referring to writing God's words on the doorposts of one's house. Assuming affixing a *mezuzah* to the resident's door does not violate facility policy, the chaplain can encourage this to be done, and perhaps even provide one for the new resident. Such a gesture certainly can also raise awareness with other staff members of the facility for the reason and importance of this practice for the Jewish resident.

An awareness of Jewish views on illness, end-of-life, dying, and death are also important. Jews do not pray as Christians pray, i.e., in the name of the Father, Son and Holy Spirit, or in the name of Jesus. It should also be understood that prayer may not be of primary importance when providing pastoral care unless the resident talks about prayer as part of his/her faith life, or requests it. At the same time, comfort and comments that can help a person cope with health issues are always helpful. It goes without saying that such comments should not include references to Christian belief or theology.

In a senior residential care facility, death, of course, is normal and inevitable. While Judaism teaches that there is definitely a life after this one, it is true that many Jews may not affirm this belief. Therefore, dying is generally not considered as "going to a better place", as some Christians believe. Nor is there an emphasis on a resurrection. The emphasis at the time of death is more on gratitude for the person's life and what the person did for the benefit of others during his/her lifetime, and sharing stories about the deceased person's relationships with family and community.

Staff members or the care facility should also be aware of certain practices that are observed when a Jewish resident dies: e.g., opening a window in the room (to allow the soul to ascend), covering all mirrors in the room (acknowledging our mortality), and calling a rabbi or Jewish chaplain. When a Jewish person dies in a non-Jewish facility, a rabbi should be called – either the person's own rabbi or one with whom arrangements have been made to provide spiritual care in the facility. A brief blessing can be said at the moment of death, a psalm can be read, or it might be appropriate for the *Shma* (Hear, O Israel; the Lord our God, the Lord is One) to be said.

While normal aftercare by the nursing staff may be performed, there is also a ritual washing and preparation of the body for burial (including the wrapping of the body in a white shroud) which is usually left to funeral home staff. If there is no Jewish funeral home in the area, the chaplain should be aware of a funeral home that handles Jewish funerals. It is a sign of respect for someone to sit with the deceased and read psalms until the funeral. Asking the family if they would like assistance in arranging for someone to do this may be quite helpful. Traditionally, as a sign of respect, Jews bury their dead as soon as possible, normally within one to three days, and in a consecrated cemetery under Jewish auspices.

It may be important to know that organ donation is not only permitted but also considered by some to be a religious obligation. In addition, sending flowers to the funeral of someone Jewish is generally not done. But a donation in memory of the person to a charity will be much appreciated by the family. Generally speaking, the purpose of the funeral is to show respect for the dead and support for the family.

At the cemetery a common Jewish tradition is for those present, if willing and able, to shovel some dirt into the grave as an act of closure and a final act of kindness for the deceased. My experience has been that if the Christian chaplain wishes to be a part of this ritual, the rabbi and family are usually (and appreciatively) accommodating.

The mourning period following the burial is called *shiva*. Traditionally it lasts seven days (shiva = seven), but may only last one, two or three days, depending on the family's wishes and practice. *Shiva* usually is held at the home of the deceased, or a family member's home. It is a time for friends to pay condolences and offer comfort, primarily by being part of a prayer service at which *Kaddish*, the traditional prayer recited by a mourner in honor and memory of a deceased loved one, is recited. It is also a time for remembering and talking – often around a table of food, as eating is a way of affirming life. Attending a *shiva* gathering is another opportunity for the Christian chaplain to extend pastoral care by greeting the family, sharing remembrances of the deceased person, and joining in the various ways that life is affirmed at a time of loss.

In addition, when the anniversary of a beloved resident's passing occurs (*yahrzeit*) the chaplain can help family members and other residents observe this milestone by offering remembrances of the deceased person, and by making sure that the tradition of lighting a memorial candle is observed. Where live candles are not permitted, electric memorial candles may be used. These may also be used during the *shiva* observance. The chaplain may want to have one or two of these electric memorial candles available for residents of the facility to use.

Another important responsibility of a chaplain in a Christian faith-based senior residential care facility is to provide education, awareness and understanding of the various religious and spiritual needs of Jewish residents to staff members who may have no prior experience with caring for people of the Jewish faith. The chaplain can be instrumental in educating other staff members, to be aware of certain words and references which may not seem appropriate, but may actually be quite offensive to residents who are Jewish. Wishing a Jewish resident Merry Christmas or Happy Easter is obviously inappropriate. Instead recognizing important Jewish holidays should be done, such as "Happy Hanukah," or "Shabbat Shalom" on the Sabbath day, or "may you have a blessed Passover." If the chaplain is involved in orientation of new staff members, this would be an ideal time to raise awareness and educate staff members. In addition, periodic in-service education sessions can raise staff members' awareness of issues that may be of specific concern for Jewish residents.

Indeed, some of these issues may often arise during the admission process itself. The admissions staff, in addition to knowing what kind of questions to ask a person/family during the admission process, can offer information about the facility that would be beneficial to the Jewish applicant and his/her family, so that an informed decision regarding admission can be made.

A prospective Jewish resident coming into a Christian facility may very well want to know about the nature of the religious activities provided in the facility. Are residents encouraged/expected to attend religious activities? Will the Jewish resident feel coerced or uncomfortable in attending? To what extent are Jewish holidays and traditions recognized and observed in the facility? Is there a rabbi on staff? May the resident's rabbi visit? Does the facility have connections with local rabbis who will make pastoral visits and conduct worship services for Jewish residents?

One important issue may be the availability of kosher food: does the dietary department have the capacity to provide kosher meals? Do staff members know about Jewish dietary laws and their importance? As part of their mandate to provide quality care, dietary and nursing staff should understand and be willing to provide food that meets a Jewish resident's dietary needs. Realizing that the kitchen of a non-Jewish facility most likely will not be equipped to provide kosher meals, it is important for staff to realize that, at a minimum, Jewish residents should not be offered pork products or shellfish. When holidays such as Passover occur, staff should also be aware of the special dietary restrictions associated with that holiday.

Yet, even with its special restrictions, Passover, as well as Hanukah, two important holidays to most Jews, can easily be observed in the facility. An important festival of the Jewish people is the annual observance of Passover, and the accompanying Seder, celebrating the liberation of the Israelites from Egypt. Most families observe the Seder at home the first and/or second night of Passover. It is customary for our facility to provide for the Jewish residents a Seder on the third night of Passover. A rabbi (or a trained lay person) usually leads the service and presides over the meal.

Each attendee is provided with an individual Seder plate to be used during the ceremony, and the menu includes traditional Jewish Seder meal foods, such as matzo-ball chicken soup, matzo-crusted baked chicken, asparagus spears, red-skinned potatoes, and a honey cake for dessert. Wine and/or grape juice are served as part of the ceremony, and other beverages are provided during the meal.

Our celebration of Hanukah, the Festival of Lights, is observed with readings and prayers accompanying the lighting of candles in the *menorah/hanukiyah*, which is placed on a stand in a common area of the facility. Stories are shared, as are treats such as cookies and candies. It is our practice to invite a Jewish resident to light one additional candle each day at sun-down during the eight days of the celebration. Again, the chaplain can provide an electric *menorah* for this observance when an open flame is prohibited, as it is in most facilities, because of fire codes and regulations.

It should also be mentioned that when there are other religious activities and services which might be attended by Jewish residents, sensitivity will hopefully lead to as much inclusiveness as possible, especially when it comes to religious language, scriptural references, and symbols. To be sure, Jewish residents may very well be uncomfortable hearing specific Christological language or seeing a cross. At the same time, if an activity in a Christian facility is planned and "advertised" as a specifically *Christian* program, religious authenticity need not be sacrificed. What is important is that the specific religious nature of the program is clear to all residents – Jewish and Christian – so that decisions can be freely made. Of course, no resident, whether cognitively able or otherwise, should be coerced or cajoled to attend, or simply "parked" in a religious program if it is not their wish to be in attendance.

If the facility is located in a large metropolitan area where there are one or more synagogues in the community, the chaplain should try to establish a relationship with one or more of the local rabbis, and arrange for periodic rabbinic visitations and the conducting of worship services for the Jewish residents. Again, in the interest of sensitivity, it is important to hold such services in a location that would be appropriate – not necessarily in the chapel where crosses and other Christian symbols are present.

Moreover, if a Jewish resident does not have a connection with a local synagogue, it is all the more incumbent upon the chaplain to keep the visiting rabbi(s) informed about such residents who may become hospitalized. Ideally, the facility will have a rabbi on staff, even only part-time, to address all of the above situations and better provide for the religious and spiritual needs of its Jewish residents. However, in the absence of rabbinic participation, laity who are knowledgeable and able to lead a worship service may do so – either a resident of the facility, or someone from the community.

Particularly, when the leading of a service is done by a family member, it can be meaningful for both resident and family. This author was privileged to be part of an experience in which a young man requested, as his *bar mitzvah* project, to assist the rabbi in leading the Shabbat services – a request readily welcomed by the rabbi. The *bar mitzvah* boy's request came because his great grandmother was a resident in our facility. He completed his project, celebrated his *bar mitzvah* at his synagogue, and then continued for several years to come to assist with the Shabbat services. Needless to say, the residents loved having him present; it helped them to feel more connected with the outside community and to also feel a sense of ongoing continuity.

I would note that in addition to our facility having good working relationships with several of the rabbis in the community, we also have a contractual arrangement with the local Jewish Federation to have the local Jewish community chaplain visit and provide services for the Jewish residents at our facility on a weekly basis. I have learned much about the faith traditions and spirituality of Jews that have enhanced my own ministry to both the Jewish and the Christian residents who live here at our facility. In addition, because of the above mentioned efforts, I have been fortunate to receive tremendous gratitude and respect from both Christian and Jewish residents and their families, and the rabbi. The experience has heightened my sensitivities and broadened my perspectives on ministry to all of God's people. I have learned that we can all "get something out of it". Indeed there is much to be gained from a shared ministry of pastoral care and love for people who are faithful to their God and to their calling to serve others through their life and faith.

Chapter 22

For You Know The Heart Of The Stranger: Addressing The Spiritual And Religious Needs Of Non-Jewish Residents In Jewish Senior Residential Care Venues

Rabbi Cary Kozberg

I n the United States, the "faith-based" focus of agencies addressing the needs of older adults is used largely to help their respective faith communities fulfill the Scriptural commandment, *You shall rise before the aged, and show deference to the old* (Leviticus 19:32). This is certainly true of those agencies that are under the auspices of Jewish communities around the country. In communities where there are Jewish Family Service agencies and/or senior residential care facilities under the auspices of the local Jewish community, the spirit of this verse and the sense of moral and religious obligation it communicates are at the heart of whatever communal resources are utilized for the physical, emotional and spiritual well-being of older adults.

Notably, juxtaposed to this verse mandating deferential treatment to older adults is another mandating that the community not only welcome strangers, but also treat them as members of the community are treated: *"The stranger who resides with you shall be to you as one of your citizens; you shall love him as yourself, for you were strangers in the land of Egypt"* (Leviticus 19:33).

Loving The Stranger

Traditional Jewish exegesis assumes that Holy Scripture, particularly the *Torah*, the five books of Moses, is of divine origin, and therefore perfect. Unlike modern scholars who approach Biblical texts from a more critical perspective, traditional Jewish exegesis has always affirmed that there are no linguistic or stylistic coincidences or accidents in the text – no unnecessary repetitions, nor is there anything "haphazard" in Scripture, or in the way it is presented. Assuming the divine origins of Scripture, adherents of this traditional approach would understand that the linking of these two commandments yields an important lesson: we are mandated to respect older adults and defer to them, *and* we are forbidden to treat them as if they were strangers. The commandment to respect the elderly includes the obligation to keep them connected to the community; we are to make sure that they are not ignored, marginalized or disenfranchised.

Among the reasons that Jewish senior residential care facilities began to proliferate after World War II, was the paramount need to help older Jews maintain their social, cultural and religious ties to Judaism and the Jewish community. In a time when there was widespread discrimination against Jews in all areas of American society, such institutions insured that older Jews (many, if not most, of whom were immigrants from Eastern Europe) could live their later years in environments that would be familiar and nurturing to them. In such environments, religious services would be available, kosher food would be served, and Jewish sacred times – Sabbath and holidays – would be honored. The ambience of these places would have a recognizably Jewish flavor. For these reasons Jewish "homes for the aged" were intended to be populated exclusively by Jews.

In recent years, changes in eligibility criteria, payor and funding sources that have impacted non-profit and proprietary care facilities, along with demographic and cultural changes within the American Jewish community itself, have led almost all Jewish-sponsored senior care facilities to rethink and revamp their admission policies to include non-Jewish residents. To be sure, such changes in admission policies at times have elicited resistance from certain quarters of the Jewish community. Given the collective memory of persecution and discrimination in times past experienced by Jews who lived in close proximity to non-Jews, it is understandable that some older Jews might react negatively to the prospect of non-Jews living among them.

However, a larger concern is often that the admission of non-Jewish residents to a Jewish senior care facility may compromise the facility's cultural and religious life, and therefore its authenticity. But even when this is not a concern, a more open admissions policy may raise a host of other questions that impact both the facility's integrity as a faith-based institution, as well as residents' individual rights. These questions may include:

- Are non-Jewish residents and their families expected to observe the Jewish dietary laws?
- Are non-Jewish residents and their families expected to observe the restrictions associated with Jewish Sabbath and other sacred holidays?
- Do Jewish religious tenets and guidelines regarding bioethical and end-of-life issues apply to non-Jewish residents of Jewish senior care facilities?
- Is the facility expected to provide for the religious/spiritual needs of non-Jewish residents as it does for its Jewish residents? And if so, to what extent?

It should be noted that every Jewish senior residential care facility is an autonomous organization that addresses these and other pertinent questions in its own way. And yet, with so many of these facilities caring for both Jewish and non-Jewish residents – sometimes with the non-Jewish census being *at least* 50% – one can assume that these questions present themselves on a frequent, if not daily basis, as administrators deal with the economic necessity of keeping beds filled. But for those who believe it is important to preserve and maintain the Jewish religious and cultural integrity of these places, these and other related questions present themselves as part of a larger ethical and religious challenge:

- How do Jewish senior residential care facilities maintain their Jewish integrity when non-Jews are part of their populations?
- Is it possible to maintain an authentic and substantive Jewish ambience, when those who are not "members of the tribe" are admitted and welcomed (and not just *tolerated*)?

As the professional who is responsible for our facility's Jewish religious and cultural ambience, I have found that not only does the presence of non-Jewish residents not compromise Jewish authenticity, but it arguably *enhances* it. Their presence may even be necessary, for admitting non-Jewish residents to a Jewish SRC is certainly a demonstrable fulfillment of the religious commandment to "welcome the stranger". In addition, Scripture makes several other references to this religious obligation[1]. The fact that this commandment is mentioned in several different places would not only affirm the importance of welcoming the stranger, but also imply the need to address lingering feelings of ethnocentric xenophobia within the Jewish community. As is clear from the biblical text, the prohibition of mistreating the stranger is based on an expected feeling of empathy, borne out of the historical Jewish experience of being outsiders: *You know the feelings of a stranger, for you were a stranger in the land of Egypt* (Exodus 23:9).

Furthermore, this core tenet is amplified by the Talmudic sages who advocated responding to misfortunes of non-Jews, along with those of their own community. Specifically, they taught that for the sake of harmonious relationships between the two communities, non-Jews who are poor must be helped; those who are sick must be visited. When necessary, it is the Jewish community's responsibility to see that they are properly buried.[2]

And lest this directive be understood as rooted only in political and "utilitarian" motives, it should be noted that proof texts for the moral and religious correctness of helping non-Jews are provided by other Scriptural references. These include: 1) the affirmation that every human being is created *b'tselem Elohim* (in the divine image)[3], and 2) the oft-repeated teaching that the *raison d'etre* of the Jewish community is to role-model Godly behavior among human beings[4] by exhibiting these attributes in their dealings with others.[5] Thus, in light of so many religious imperatives regarding how older persons and strangers are to be treated, it is possible to deduce that welcoming non-Jewish elderly into a Jewish SRC amplifies the obligation.

What might a non-Jewish resident expect when coming to live in a Jewish SRC? To be sure, it depends on how the term "Jewish SRC" is understood. If the facility is "Jewish" because most or all of its residents are Jews, but the facility's programming includes few, if any, expressions

---

[1]   See Exodus 12.48, 23.9 and 23.20; Deuteronomy 10.19 among others.

[2]   Talmud Gittin 61a; see also Maimonides, Mishneh Torah, *Hilchot Melachim*, chapter 10 (end).

[3]   Genesis 1.27.

[4]   Genesis 18.19; Isaiah 43.10.

[5]   See Deuteronomy 11.22, 28.9 and Isaiah 42.6 ff.

of Jewish religion and culture (i.e. Jewish holidays are not celebrated, Jewish dietary laws are not followed, Jewish cultural programs are rare), then a non-Jewish resident might find it easier to fit in more quickly.

However, if the facility is "Jewish" in more than its census, if it is a place where Jewish people not only live, but also a place where Jewish religious practice and ethical tenets inform and guide almost every aspect of life – from the quality of care and the kinds of activities offered to relationships among residents, family and staff – then the non-Jewish resident might find his/her acclimation a bit more challenging.

As mentioned above, questions regarding expectations of non-Jewish residents' participation in Jewish practices do not have universal responses; each Jewish facility is an autonomous institution. Even with input from rabbis and other sources, solutions to any given issue may vary from facility to facility. What follows is a description of how Wexner Heritage Village (WHV), a Jewish SRC in Columbus, Ohio with a 35-40% non-Jewish census, has addressed the challenge of meeting the spiritual/religious needs of its non-Jewish residents, while maintaining an authentically Jewish religious and cultural ambience.

"Tolerance Is Practiced Here"

From the day that our first non-Jewish resident came through our doors over 15 years ago, the attitude of our professional and lay leadership to admitting non-Jews has generally reflected the religious and ethical tenets mentioned above. To be sure, there were one or two "ethno-centrics" from the community whose responses initially were less than gracious, but these were in no way taken seriously by the rest of the administration and board. I believe that this was largely due to the fact that WHV had – and continues to have – a "faith-based" Jewish ethos that is well-established, robust and ubiquitous. For this reason admitting non-Jews into a facility that had heretofore been "all Jewish", posed little if any threat.

At the same time, knowing the kinds of difficulties that Jewish residents sometimes face in SRCs where staff are unfamiliar with and/or unsympathetic to their needs, we wanted our "new folks" to feel as comfortable and as acclimated as possible. Happily, as our non-Jewish population has grown, the spirit of openness, tolerance, and discernment has grown as well. Indeed, this is reflected in the increased resources over the years devoted to meeting the spiritual and religious needs of these individuals.[6]

For example, when there were only two or three non-Jewish residents in our long-term care facility out of a total census of 200, Christian clergy might agree to conduct worship and offer pastoral visits on a volunteer basis. However, this arrangement had limited success. As the population grew, we contracted with Lutheran Social Services for regular weekly visits from a pastor, in addition to weekly visits from the Catholic priest in whose parish our facility is located. Presently, a full-time Christian chaplain is part of our Religious Life Department. In addition to conducting two weekly worship services (one for our cognitively-intact residents, and one for those who are cognitively impaired), she makes pastoral visits, counsels with families and staff, and also arranges pastoral visits by priests and Eucharistic ministers for our Catholic residents.

In this way, all of our residents have opportunities to continue their religious and spiritual lives, according to the faith traditions which they affirm. For the sake of residents' dignity, they are not automatically taken to a religious program "just to give them something to do," nor are they assisted to any worship service unless they wish to attend. Staff members are careful not to bring Jewish residents to Christian worship, and vice-versa, unless the residents expressly ask to attend. To be sure, we have found that non-Jewish residents often appreciate the opportunity to attend – and participate in – Jewish worship services and other specifically Jewish religious programs. (Indeed, over the years there have been several who have attended more faithfully than their fellow Jewish residents!)

It should be noted that when it comes to welcoming and helping non-Jewish residents to acclimate to the ambience of a Jewish SRC, the challenges are certainly not all on "the Jewish side". Moving into a Jewish SRC with a robustly Jewish ethos, non-Jewish residents and their families frequently have a lot with which to become acquainted, particularly if their experience with Jews and Judaism has been limited.

For this reason, our Admissions Department usually discusses a few of the "basics" with new residents and their families, Jewish and non-Jewish alike. Admissions staff are careful to remind them that our facility is a Jewish "faith-based" institution, that Jewish religious

---

6   As of this writing, all non-Jewish residents of WHV who list a religious preference have, with a handful of exceptions, identified as Christians (either Roman Catholic or belonging to a Protestant denomination).

practice and culture is a major part of life in the facility, and that certain aspects with which they will come into regular contact, i.e. the Jewish dietary laws (*kashrut*) need to be remembered and respected. Our admissions materials state that 1) all food served to residents is prepared according to the Jewish dietary laws, 2) all public areas in the building are "kosher" areas, and 3) food brought into the facility is permitted ONLY in residents' private rooms, or designated "non-kosher" eating areas.

Because keeping the Sabbath and observing holidays is a staple of Jewish religious life, new residents and their families are also made aware of those Sabbath/holiday restrictions which are part of Jewish life at WHV. They are informed that on these days, regularly scheduled occurrences – i.e. baths, therapies, etc. – will be shifted away from those times when worship is scheduled; they are informed that on these sacred days regular admissions and discharges usually do not take place (except in unavoidable circumstances), and that Administrative offices are closed and regular business is suspended. In addition, we communicate to all new residents and their families that our responses to end-of-life issues are grounded in the belief that *every* person is created in the image of God, regardless of his/her physical condition, and that our care for residents at the end of their lives reflects that belief, regardless of their religious beliefs.

One could assume that so many of these "unusual" conditions or limitations which are not a part of the culture of other SRCs, would lead to complaints from many non-Jewish residents and their families. On the contrary, with the exception of some residents/families who may have some difficulty getting used to certain ethnic Jewish foods (gefilte fish is indeed an acquired taste), or not fully understanding some of the restrictions of *kashrut* (i.e. regarding outside food in the public areas), our experience has generally been that non-Jewish residents and their families usually respect our need to preserve our Jewish religious and cultural integrity. Indeed, not only do they understand and respect it, but they also very much appreciate it because they know that the high quality of care is itself a manifestation of a commitment to our Jewish religious teachings. They understand that our commitment to proper caring for those who are frail and vulnerable is intertwined with Jewish religious commitments, and that they all come from the same Source.

With this understanding, non-Jewish residents and families also appreciate our helping them to increase their own awareness and understanding of Jewish traditions, rituals and celebrations. They know that they are always welcome to attend any and all Jewish worship services and religious programs if they so choose – and many do! In addition, our non-Jewish residents soon learn that, in such an atmosphere, their respect of Jewish traditions and religious life will be reciprocated. Knowing that there is a Christian chaplain on staff who provides regularly scheduled worship and Scripture study, they also will be able to continue to practice their own faith traditions.

Thus, while our non-Jewish residents may be in the minority, numerically speaking, they are still important members of our community. Observances of American holidays such as Independence Day and Thanksgiving are planned with all residents in mind, as is our resident memorial service, which includes Scriptural selections and poetry which everyone can comfortably read or recite. Indeed, the experience of feeling part of our community is nowhere more affirmed than in this monthly gathering. Over and over again, family members of non-Jewish residents have expressed their appreciation for how we cared for their loved ones, but also how we continued to demonstrate that care by honoring their memories after they had died.

The December Dilemma

Even with our attempts to affirm cultural and religious diversity, there is one sensitive issue that annually presents a potential challenge to maintaining that fine balance between our commitment to tolerance and diversity, and our commitment to an authentic Jewish ambience: the observance of Christmas. I say "potential challenge" because, thus far, our Jewish facility has succeeded in providing opportunities for those residents and families who celebrate the Christmas holiday, without compromising our Jewish identity and sense of authenticity. Over the years, our success has largely been because of the following policy:

- During the December holiday season, *all* residents have the right to enhance / decorate their rooms however they choose – as long as the decorations are *inside* their rooms, which are considered private domains. (All of our rooms are all single occupancy.)

- Because the front side of residents' room doors face the public areas, residents are respectfully requested (and expected) to refrain from putting holiday decorations on the front of their doors.[7]

And yet, even as we navigate every December through potentially troubled waters, a tremendous source of pride for our Jewish facility is our annual resident/family Christmas worship service and party which we have hosted for over a decade. The pride is rooted not only in the knowledge that we are providing for the religious needs of our Christian residents and their families, but also in the fact that the party and reception following the worship service, is prepared in our kitchen, and is therefore *kosher!* A kosher Christmas party![8] What better way can be found to demonstrate that specific Jewish ritual obligations can be fulfilled without compromising the ethical obligation to make "the stranger" feel welcome! With this in mind, I am always pleased to begin this particular program every year with a word of welcome and appreciation for the spirit of tolerance and diversity that this program represents.

Another Challenge To Religious Integrity

At times other situations arise which present challenges not necessarily to the religious integrity of the facility, but to my own religious integrity as a rabbi and a Jew. As a trained chaplain, I am prepared to meet people "where they are" – to listen to their concerns and situation, while respecting and trying to understand the particular spirituality or belief system with which they live in the world. At the same time, I am grounded in my own particular spirituality and belief system which provide the resources from which I draw in my roles as

---

7   This policy is similar to the one governing the observance of the Jewish dietary laws: private rooms and private offices are not under kosher restrictions, while food served and eaten in all public areas (resident dining areas, living areas, etc.) must be kosher. In addition, our staff dining room and other designated "non-kosher" areas are "open", with no Jewish dietary restrictions. These solutions have worked for all concerned, primarily because they are based on mutual respect and a serious concern and understanding for everyone's needs.

8   My co-editor James Michaels is proud that the Hebrew Home of Greater Washington offers the world's only kosher-for-Passover Easter dinner.

rabbi and a chaplain.

In the professional world of clinical chaplaincy, there are those who believe that chaplains should be prepared to do whatever is necessary to meet the religious and spiritual needs of the people they encounter, even if that entails compromising or violating the chaplain's own religious principles and beliefs. This approach to chaplaincy maintains that at times Jewish chaplains should be prepared to remove their *kipot/* skullcaps, or pray "in the name of Jesus" with believing Christians, and Christian chaplains who believe every prayer must be offered "in the name of Jesus" should be prepared to forego this requirement if necessary.

I do not advocate that position! While I am committed to flexibility (most of this chapter has focused on flexibility in action), I believe that to be an effective rabbi and chaplain, one has to be *authentic*, both personally and professionally. I believe that my chaplaincy is based on my rabbinic calling; thus, to practice chaplaincy any other way would, for me, be inauthentic. As a member of the clergy, when I meet with a non-Jewish resident or family member and the opportunity for a pastoral encounter occurs, I will listen to, pray and counsel with, teach and explain, or just offer a "ministry of presence".

But I also believe such a presence must be one totally authentic to what and who I am: that is the only way I as a rabbi and chaplain can hope to represent God's authentic Presence.[9] In this way, authenticity can be more important than which religious faith I represent. It also means that I must recognize the same need for, and right to, authenticity in others. So, when someone needs or requests prayer and pastoral care that is specifically out of the Christian tradition, I will connect them with our Christian chaplain, or contact the person's own clergy. Even when there are acknowledged religious differences, I have found that my response is nevertheless appreciated because people in need usually appreciate an empathy born out of authenticity that reaches across religious differences. In my experience, authenticity eclipsing religious differences has manifested itself in at least two ways:

1) we have non-Jewish residents regularly attending our Jewish worship services and Torah study, and

2) the families of non-Jewish residents often feel comfortable

---

9   For more on authenticity in chaplaincy, see "The Chaplain as an Authentic and Ethical Presence" by David Zucker, T. Patrick Bradley, and Bonita Taylor, in *Chaplaincy Today*, Vol. 23. No. 2.

asking me to conduct, or participate in, the funeral services of their loved ones.

But the real power of how religious authenticity can eclipse religious differences became apparent to me several years ago after a High Holiday service at which Hattie was present. Hattie was an African-American lady who, before she passed on, was a regular attendee at our Sabbath and Holiday services. A student of Scripture and church-going lady all her life, Hattie resonated to good preaching. She knew what it meant to be truly inspired and uplifted by a well-delivered sermon. When the service concluded, she came up to me, looked me in straight in the eye and said, "Raaabi (sic) ... your sermon ... that was RIGHTEOUS!!" In my thirty-plus years as a rabbi, I have never felt so good about a compliment. Moreover, I was pleased that our connection was so close – that, even though she was a believing Christian and I am a believing Jew, I was truly "her rabbi", and she wanted me to know that. (On a more personal note: her memory has a special place in my heart, and her photo still adorns my office.)

Experiences such as these are reminders that while religious and spiritual differences among those who reside and work in senior residential care facilities need to be acknowledged and certain boundaries must be respected, the words of the prophet Malachi continue to be a touchstone: "Have we not all one Father? Has not one God created us?"[10] In our facility, as we continue to respond to the needs of *all* of our residents, the answer to both of these questions continues to be "Yes!"

---

10   Malachi 2.10.

Part Three ~ What Will The Future Bring

Chapter 23

The Future Of Senior Residential Care In America

Scott Janco

January 1, 2011, was hailed as the date when the oldest Baby Boomers became "senior citizens." The years ahead will see an exponential increase of Americans over the age of 65. It can be anticipated that the numbers of people receiving senior residential health care will also increase dramatically. *Leading Age,* formerly the American Association of Homes and Services for the Aging (AAHSA), estimates that by 2020, 12 million older Americans will require either community-based or residential care.

With this projected elderly population growth, and a growing demand for services, the real issues will focus on how we as a society will meet the needs for senior residential care and what changes will be needed to deliver those services. Consider these general facts, also provided by *Leading Age.*[1]

According to most recent data, more than 1.7 million Americans live in skilled nursing facilities. Almost another 1 million people live in assisted living residences.

There are more than 1.1 million seniors in some type of senior housing community in the United States.

An estimated 44.4 million Americans (21% of all adults in the U.S.) provide unpaid care to another adult age 18 or older.

90% of individuals who receive care at home receive help from family and friends, and 80% rely solely on these individuals for assistance.

---

1   www.leadingage.org

Divided into four sections, this chapter will focus on the challenges that result from these facts. The first will discuss the history of the senior residential care system and how it has evolved from the beginning of our nation. Understanding its history, and that of the welfare system, will not only help us understand implications for our current system but also help us discern the trends for the future. Indeed, as we will see, some of the current trends are very similar to the past.

Second, we will look at how the 2010 Patient Protection and Affordable Care Act could affect the financing and delivery of senior residential care.

The third section will explore how elder care has historically been financed, and how this has played a pivotal role in how senior residential care is delivered.

Finally, we will discuss the leading future trends for service delivery: the changing roles of nursing homes, the growing trend toward assisted living and home and community based services, as well as the role of family as caregivers and key decision makers for elderly relatives.

Senior Residential Care In America: A Brief History

The Post-Revolution Years

The beginnings of senior residential care can be traced back to colonial America. In the late 1700s, the United States was a "young persons'" country. Life expectancy was shorter due to high infant and childhood mortality rates, and the majority of the population was comprised of European immigrants. Crossing the ocean by ship was very difficult and very few elderly people attempted it. In addition, Africans who were brought to this country as slaves also tended to be young.

Security in old age meant having a family and/or property. Children took care of their elderly parents and it was expected that families took care of their own. If an elderly person had wealth, he could hire help. Those without wealth or family to help were dependent on public welfare or charity care.

The public welfare system at that time was based on the English Poor Laws. Basically, these laws legislated that it was the government's responsibility to provide for those who could not care for themselves, leaving the details to local officials.[2] Initially, the indigent were given

---

2   History of Long Term Care, www.elderweb.com/home/book, page 3

cash payments to live on. Eventually, the cost of this type of program was deemed too expensive for local governments, so poorhouses or almshouses for welfare recipients were built. This solution was believed to be a more cost effective way to care for the indigent. Eventually, poorhouses attracted anyone who could not live on their own, and this included poor dependent elderly.

The 19th Century

There were three important factors that shaped the history of senior care in this country: the role of the family, the role of wealth in hiring others to provide care, and the beginning of government involvement in financing senior residential care. The 1800s saw America growing rapidly and families beginning to disperse throughout the nation. Children moved from farms to the cities to find work, or to western territories where land was cheaper in order to set up their own farms. In 1800, the largest cities were all in the thirteen original colonies. By 1850, however, cities like Cincinnati, St. Louis, and New Orleans grew to be larger than these eastern cities. Over time, the westward migration made it less likely that children would automatically live close enough to their parents to provide them care in their later years.

As children moved away, their parents often ended up in poorhouses when they got older. This caused an increase in the population of these places in the early part of the 19th century. The living conditions in most were deplorable and the government agencies charged with running the poorhouses often did as little as possible to keep costs down. Over time, the system itself came under scrutiny. Dorthea Dix reported finding women chained and kept in pens in some poorhouses. Frail elderly people were frightened, and sometimes injured other inmates with whom they were forced to share rooms, including criminals, alcoholics or patients who were insane.[3] In response to concerns about abuse and filthy living conditions, some states set up oversight boards that were supposed to inspect, control, and report on poorhouse conditions and operations. Their efforts led to some improvement of conditions, with the most significant change being the separation of sane residents from those who were insane, and the dependent elderly from the able-bodied. Another sign of progress was the passage of new laws that allowed charitable organizations to operate like corporations. These new not-

---

3   Ibid., page 9

for-profit organizations started building homes for the elderly to avoid the squalor of the poorhouses. Although they were modest, they were lavish when compared to the poorhouses.

Another important development of the 19th century was the appearance of hospitals and chronic care facilities. Hospitals have some historical ties to the poorhouse system, as do nursing homes. In the early 1800s, hospitals were not places where people could be cured, but rather where people went to die. Fortunately, in the last half of the century, medicine as a science started to understand the nature and causes many diseases, and as an art started to move away from its "Dark Ages" procedures, and develop more effective and reliable methods.

Nursing also emerged as a distinct profession in the late 19th century, along with that of home health care. Hospitals needed nurses to care for their patients and began to create schools to train them. Wealthier families sometimes hired them to care for their invalid and elderly members. Although families with fewer means could not afford private nurses, this was also the time that home care for the poor began to appear.[4]

In addition, the Civil War left thousands of disabled veterans in need of senior residential care. Although the devastating impact of the war caused veterans benefits to be expanded,[5] the cash assistance was not enough for some veterans and their families. This led the federal government to begin to build hospitals and homes to provide to provide for the needs of these veterans.

In 1875, American Express developed the first private employer-sponsored pension program. The Baltimore and Ohio Railroad started its pension program in 1884 and its model was soon followed by other railroads.[6] These pensions did not require employees to contribute but usually required the employee to have very long tenure – as long as thirty years – to collect any benefits.

The 19th century also saw the beginning of planned communities and retirement campuses. Sailor's Snug Harbor was built 1822 on Staten Island New York as a 130-acre campus for "old and worn out seamen." It was continuously in operation until the late 1960s.[7]

---

4   Ibid., page 20
5   Ibid., page 21
6   Ibid., page 22
7   Ibid., page 17

The Early 20th Century

The early part of the 20th century saw a continuing development and improvement of the health and welfare systems in this country. Hundreds of volunteer-run and not-for-profit old age homes were built in the late 1800s and early 1900s. As the population grew, more buildings were added to campuses, including hospitals and staff quarters, and the campuses themselves began to resemble small towns.

As the health care system improved, the number of people reaching old age increased dramatically. The average life expectancy increased by 10 years from 1900 to 1930 and another 15 years from 1930 to 1990.[8] Since fewer people succumbed to death during childhood, a larger percentage of the population was able to survive into their later years.

During this time, the United States changed from being a largely agrarian society to one that was mostly urban. At the beginning of the 19th century, 40% of the population lived in the cities; by 1900 that percentage had increased to 75%. Many new city dwellers came from rural areas, while others were from the multitude of immigrants entering the country, most of whom came from Europe.

The cities' continued growth caused them to experience "urban sprawl". The rich could afford to escape by building houses away from the congestion of the city centers. Many of the less well-off, including the burgeoning immigrant classes, moved into the city's existing housing structures, and thus tenements were created.

Moreover, at this time the structure and size of families was changing. Urban families were much smaller than rural families. On the farm, a large family was an economic asset: children were expected to help with the daily chores of farming. In the city, this wasn't the case. In the city, having children meant additional mouths to feed. Although some sold newspapers or shined shoes on the streets to bring in money to help their families, they could not contribute support that was significant until they graduated or quit school. Since living in the city made it economically disadvantageous to have a large family, family size began to shrink.[9]

---

8   Ibid., page 25, 26.

9   It should be noted that the impact of this trend will continue far into the future. Seniors may come to outnumber younger citizens, and one result will be that the income, tax payments, and/or gifts to charity of the latter may be insufficient to provide for care for the former.

City-dwellers usually were not self-employed and the working class among them often had jobs that required physical strength and endurance which could not be done indefinitely. Blue collar workers whose physical abilities waned were terminated. For the first time, older Americans faced the prospect of being unemployed.

As those without families to rely on became unable to support themselves, some states began to provide public assistance to the impoverished elderly. Most of these elderly assistance laws were limited. The state helped finance the cost of assistance only for those who had no other income, and only if counties enacted elderly pension laws to contribute to the overall costs.

The 20th century saw more employers participating in pension plan programs. In 1896, New Jersey created the first state-sponsored pension plan for teachers. From 1900 to 1903 real progress was made for older Americans who were not disabled or in need and more private companies began providing retirement plans. In 1911, the first pension program for all state government employees was instituted in Massachusetts. In 1920, the Civil Service Retirement Act created a retirement system for many government employees.[10] Retirement plans meant older adults had some means of paying for senior residential care.

Government Involvement In Senior Care

The Great Depression had a tremendous impact on the lives of Americans, but especially on those who were older. Family life and work conditions significantly changed in some regions of the country, as almost half of the working age population became unemployed. Retirees or those close to retirement saw their lifetime savings vanish. Most were not well enough to work and those who were healthy were unable to find jobs that would allow them to recoup their life savings. These individuals became completely dependent on their families, but the prevailing economic conditions drained the resources of younger family members, so that there was little left to help their parents.

In 1935, Congress passed the Social Security Act that created a national old-age assistance program. Title I, called Old Age Assistance (OAA), provided cash payments to poor elderly citizens, regardless of their work history, and provided for a federal government match of state old-age assistance expenditures. OAA is an important item in the history

---

10   Ibid., page 30

of senior residential care because it was the predecessor of the current Medicaid program, the primary funding source for long-term care.

Title II established a fund for workers, the monies of which would be used to care for them in old age. Workers contributed to this fund while still working. Worker contributions were to be matched by contributions from employers, but without government financial input. Since it's inception, Title II has become one of the main sources of income for the elderly and is the part of the Social Security Act with which most Americans are familiar.

A major debate before passage of the Social Security Act focused on how to provide support to the impoverished elderly while eliminating the poorhouse system. One suggestion was to give these individuals cash payments – called "pensions" – that would hopefully make it easier for them to remain in their own homes, and thus discourage them from turning to poorhouses for assistance.[11] Another concern regarding the help provided by poorhouses was its cost. It was believed that cash payments to the needy elderly to help them remain in their own homes would be half the cost of going to an institution.

After much debate it was decided to structure OAA to prohibit federal matching funds for any payment to residents of public institutions or poorhouses. This prohibition of federal dollars to public institutions that cared for the elderly stimulated the need for private nursing homes. Initially, these payments to proprietary nursing homes were not sufficient, forcing some elderly to find shared accommodations in order to make do. Others required various levels of nursing care or just could not live on their own. One consequence was that choosing to go to a poorhouse would mean a loss of benefits.

At the time, most not-for-profit homes for the aged were sponsored by religious or fraternal groups, and thus admission was restricted to members of their sponsoring organizations. This was done for financial reasons; these homes relied on their memberships for donations to support their operations, and could not afford to meet the needs of those who were not members of their faith group or fraternal organization. Hence, for-profit nursing homes began to proliferate.

During World War II construction and development of nursing homes ceased throughout the country, and by the end of the war, the buildings of many already in existence needed renovation or replacement. Of particular concern, was the quality of the country's

---

11   Ibid., page 38

health care infrastructure. It was believed that improvement would come only by dedicating substantial funds to build and renovate hospitals. The Hill-Burton Act of 1946 created a system to provide federal funds for the construction of new hospitals and the renovation of existing facilities. The act allowed not-for-profit hospitals to access funding as loans which would be repaid by providing a certain amount of free care to the needy.[12]

An unforeseen result of Hill-Burton was the conversion of many old hospitals into nursing homes. Because post-war demand for construction made it hard to find sufficient resources to build new buildings, many older buildings – including hotels and private residences were converted to nursing homes. Because they were financed through Hill-Burton, they were designated as "not-for-profit".

In 1950, amendments to the Social Security Act allowed state governments to pay providers directly for services. This was a significant change in the way public welfare resources were delivered and paid for. With nursing homes contracting directly with state governments for payment, they began to receive a new and more reliable source of revenue. In order to raise expected standards of care, these amendments also required states receiving federal matching funds to create licensure systems and standards for nursing homes and hospitals.

The 1959 Housing Act created a program called Section 202. This program provided low-interest loans for construction to those not-for-profit organizations that provided housing for the elderly. Section 202 buildings could provide congregate meals, housekeeping, personal care, social work, and transportation for medical appointments and social activities to their residents. Many faith-based and fraternal organizations used this funding to add independent living apartments near their old age homes, creating campuses which were named "continuous care retirement communities."[13] This program was administered by the Federal Housing Administration (FHA) and the Small Business Administration (SBA).

All of this new activity made developers and lenders more aware of the industry, with additional financing coming in from private sources, even for projects not covered by federal guarantees. The new construction activity benefited developers more than it did the public. Nursing homes built with FHA or SBA funds were not subject to the

---

12   Ibid., page 47
13   Ibid., page 60

medical standards and criteria spelled out in Hill-Burton. Moreover, nursing homes built with private financing did not have to meet federal standards of care. Consequently, problems related to quality of care in these nursing homes increased dramatically.

In 1964, one of Lyndon Johnson's presidential campaign promises was to implement a national health insurance program for the elderly called Medicare. There was much debate about this program and strong opposition came from the American Medical Association. In order for the program to be enacted by Congress, all of the concepts proposed regarding health insurance for the elderly were incorporated into amendments to the Social Security Act in 1965, which established the Medicare and Medicare programs. It was not long before the cost of both programs quickly exceeded expectations.

Finally, there is the last major innovation regarding senior residential care, namely assisted living. Assisted living facilities have evolved over the past two decades and are rapidly becoming a popular alternative to nursing homes. Assisted living has emerged as an option on the continuum of care for people who cannot live independently, but who do not need the 24-hour medical care provided by nursing homes. Most assisted living facilities offer residents their own private apartment or room, and provide assistance with activities of daily living (ADL), such as medication administration, personal care services, and monitoring residents' activities to ensure their health, safety, and well being.[14]

The Patient Protection and Affordable Care Act (Health Care Reform)

Since 2009, there has been much written about health care reform. Even though the Patient Protection and Affordable Care Act was passed in 2010, it is still the subject of much debate; as of this writing, there are attempts to curtail its provisions or repeal it entirely. While space does not permit a full discussion of all of the provisions affecting senior residential care and their impact on providers and beneficiaries (such a discussion would surely take several hundred pages), one aspect of

---

14   The above history is admittedly brief, and there is much that has not been included. Those elements that were included are the ones that will have the biggest impact on the future of senior residential care and how it is delivered. As we will see, much of its future is really part of its past.

the act deserves special attention because it was the first attempt by the federal government to address the increasing need for a systematic approach to paying for senior residential care. The fact that it won't be implemented does not diminish the need for such an approach.

The Affordable Care Act, as passed, contained the Community Living Assistance Services and Support Act (or CLASS Act). It established the nation's first government-sponsored program of senior residential care insurance. Enrollment could begin as early as age 18, and it provided a guaranteed daily benefit of $50 when a person became disabled or required residential care. What may be of greatest significance is that it allowed these payments to be made to family members who, though untrained, served as primary caregivers for individuals living at home who needed the assistance.

According to an article by accountant Rachel Lee,[15] inclusion of this provision recognized that current practices in the payment and provision of care will not be adequate in the future. Indeed, as the baby boomers age, the care needs and demands of the disabled and elderly, along with the economic situation the nation will face in the next few decades, make the necessity of finding ways to provide services as efficiently as possible an immediate and serious one.

As Lee points out, the CLASS Act was the beginning of a movement away from the institutionalized "spend-down" approach to caring for the nation's elderly, and toward providing working adults the opportunity to plan for their future senior residential care needs. It provided some relief to caregivers who are currently unpaid, and acted as a supplement to existing insurance. In addition, its cash benefit encouraged innovation among entrepreneurs and providers of non-medical services and supports. The plan could have been used to offset costs in more traditional care settings. However, like other reform initiatives, its focus was to change the system to which Americans have grown accustomed and thereby promote a more independent life for the aging and disabled populations.

In October 2011, the Obama administration announced it was suspending work on implementing the CLASS Act because "it would not work." Despite this fact, it seems likely that the government will continue to shift payments heretofore allocated for institutionalized care and direct them to cover care provided at home. Howard Gleckman has identified many new community-based projects which will augment

---

15   Cf. "CLASS act" on the website www.leadingage.org

publicly funded care for the elderly who remain at home.[16] Given the desire of most seniors not to move into skilled nursing facilities, as well as the potential for saving public funds, this trend is likely to remain the preferred option for both individuals and government agencies. Organizations which advocate for senior care, such as *Leading Age*, have continued to press for work to continue on the CLASS Act, or something similar.

Financing Senior Residential Care

Since the late 1700s, finding ways to pay for the senior residential care of the poor and destitute has been an ongoing challenge for American society. If we compare circumstances at the time of our nation's beginning to today, the similarities are striking. At that time and up to the present, the wealthy could hire servants to take care of them. Today, affluent elders can employ private duty health care workers, or afford the senior residential care accommodations of their choice. For others, children or members of the extended family were expected to provide care. Today, baby boomers often take on the role of primary caregiver for an elderly parent, while others help their parents pay for senior residential care. The poor elderly of the 1700s who did not have family to care for them went to the poorhouse. In the present day, the elderly who have exhausted their life savings, do not have family who can take care of them and need care, usually end up in a nursing home, paid for by Medicaid.

To be sure, the similarities do not include the conditions or quality of care. The conditions in modern nursing homes are infinitely better than those of the poorhouses. What is similar, however, is the financing. Poorhouses were funded through local and county taxes. According to AAHSA, tax monies in the form of Medicaid pay for 49% of all senior residential care spending. The point is that just as in the past, senior residential care continues to be financed through government sources.

---

16   Howard Gleckman, *Caring for our Parents* (2009). See especially chapters 6 and 13. Editor's note: In private conversation, Gleckman noted that even if the CLASS Act had been implemented, there would have been many challenges to its full implementation. To wit, states are not mandated to make Medicaid payments for home-based care. Given the current political movement to reduce government spending, there might not have been sufficient designated funds to cover home care for seniors, or ancillary services like meals-on-wheels or wheel chair-accessible public transportation – JM.

And as our population continues to age, more elderly will rely on Medicaid to pay for their senior residential care needs, which will place more of a burden on an already constrained financing mechanism.

For years now, Medicaid spending has been under scrutiny, and health care policy makers continue to try to find ways to curtail Medicaid spending. Perhaps the real issue is not *how much* we spend on Medicaid but rather *how* we spend it; in other words perhaps the real question is not one of "quantity" but of "quality". One way to better control Medicaid expenses is to develop a system that promotes preventive care, wellness, and chronic disease management, with a built-in mechanism for managing costs. One model that does all of this with a per person capitation rate is PACE (described below).

Finally, the last item dealing with the financing of senior residential care – and one that needs immediate intention – is affordable housing for low to moderate income elderly. *Leading Age/AAHSA* estimates there are more than 300,000 units of Section 202 affordable senior housing available, but the demand greatly exceeds the availability: The problem will likely become much larger and more serious as the elderly population exceeds 71 million by 2030.

Future Trends For Service Delivery

On the other hand, the good news is that most of the components of the future delivery model for senior residential care are already in place. In fact, some have been around for many years. What will change are the roles these components will play and what their significance will be in the emerging senior residential care market. At present, many of these changes are, and will continue to be dictated by the prospective residents and in many cases, their adult children.

Thus, to better understand these changes we need to understand the senior residential care market and how it is changing. Americans are living longer and are generally in better health than previous generations. The "65 years and older" population is expected to number more than 71 million by 2026. Currently, the fastest growing segment of the population is comprised of people 85 years and older. The longevity and better health among Americans is due in large part to advancements in medicine, better technology, and better pharmaceuticals. Moreover, as their age expectancy and health standards have risen, so have Americans' expectations regarding their quality of life. Indeed, it is these expectations that are driving the senior residential care industry's response of offering creative alternatives to the traditional nursing home.

The increasing participatory role of family members as care providers and key decision makers will certainly be of consequence to future service delivery. It is becoming more common for middle-aged children to assume the role of caregivers for an elderly parent, even if they live a long distance away, and also more common for parents to move across country to be near their adult children. Often it is the adult children who find the appropriate housing for their parents usually within minutes of their homes.[17]

Another emerging trend is home- and community-based services. Many older adults are choosing to remain in their homes rather than to move into some form of senior housing. This trend is being driven in part by a change in federal government policy. Until very recently, eligibility for Medicaid required that a senior citizen had to deplete all assets to qualify for Medicaid assistance in receiving nursing home care. Now the government provides matching funds to states that provide service to the elderly, which are used primarily to allow low-income elderly persons to remain in their homes. This approach was used successfully in the 1960s to try to control Medicaid costs. Today, the same need exists, and it will certainly grow as the number of indigent elderly increases.

Another important program designed to help the elderly remain in their homes is the Program of All-inclusive Care for the Elderly (PACE). The PACE philosophy asserts that it is better for the well-being of seniors with chronic care needs and their families to be served in the community whenever possible.[18] PACE programs are sponsored by local not-for-profit agencies, which receive a blended Medicare and Medicaid monthly capitation rate. The PACE agency is responsible for addressing all of their participants' health care needs, including physician care, hospitalization, nursing home care, home care services, and prescription drugs. Those who are not eligible for Medicaid can

---

17   The severe economic downtown of 2008-2011 has resulted in another trend. Anecdotal evidence indicates that as some adult children have lost their jobs, they have brought their aging parents into their homes and have begun serving as their primary caregivers. It remains to be seen how long this trend lasts and whether it will have an enduring impact on the delivery of care to the elderly.

18   National PACE Association Web Site www.npaonline.org/website

participate in a PACE program by paying the Medicaid portion of the blended rate. The real advantage of this program is that it delivers high quality services and care for a predictable cost. Unfortunately, despite its excellence and affordability, PACE has thus far not been successful in attracting great numbers; its current number is only about 25,000 participants. It is hoped that as its numbers increase, it will be a model for future care of the frail elderly and chronically ill.[19]

As mentioned earlier, assisted living continues to emerge as an important and popular segment in the elder care continuum. Individuals in need of assistance with activities of daily living, but not skilled care continue to seek assisted-living options over nursing home care. Today's health care consumers and their families want accommodations that are less institutional, with more privacy, and in a dignified and home-like setting.

During the last decade, the increase in the number of these facilities and units has been particularly strong, with 60% of the assisted-living units built between 1995 and 2001. According to its most recent data, *Leading Age* estimates that nearly 1 million people live in assisted living residences.

With the fastest growing age segment of the population consisting of those 85 years and older, the frequency of Alzheimer's Disease among Americans will increase. Statistics from The Alzheimer's Association indicate that 42% of the population 85 and older and 19% of individuals 75 to 84 years old have some form of dementia.[20] Additionally, more than 50 percent of residents in assisted living facilities and nursing homes have some form of dementia or cognitive impairment. The U.S. Census Bureau's 2004 interim projections estimate by 2030, there will be 9.6 million Americans 85 years or older. Based on the Alzheimer's Association estimate, four million of them will have some form of dementia. This certainly will have a major impact on the senior residential care industry.

Looking into the future, perhaps the most significant change to be expected will be the role of nursing homes. Since the 1950s, nursing homes have been the mainstay for senior residential care. Most were

---

19   The PACE program offers many more benefits and would take several chapters to describe. To learn more about PACE and all of it benefits, contact the National PACE Association in Alexandria, VA.

20   Alzheimer Association, "Alzheimer's Disease Facts and Figures, 2008.

designed to resemble acute care hospitals consisting of nursing stations and semi-private rooms with a shared bathroom. Meals were brought to the nursing units on trays, and residents were bathed in communal bathing facilities.

Such accommodations are appropriate for acute care hospitals. The typical patient stay is short, usually three to six days, and most patients can tolerate such accommodations for a few days. Yet even hospitals themselves are moving away from this model.[21] Today, residents and potential residents of senior residential care and their families want accommodations that are more dignified, more private, and reflect a more home-like atmosphere. Because a person who moves into a senior residential care center may expect to live there for several years, the desire for privacy is understandable. Moreover, as nursing facilities market their facilities, they are increasingly being encouraged to cater to the tastes of adult children as well. Amenities like having high speed Internet connection available may not mean much to their 85-year-old mother, but may very significant to her children.

In the future, skilled nursing facilities will not be the "homes for aged" that they once were, but rather the last stop on the continuum of senior residential care. As seniors remain in their own homes for longer periods of time, or choose to move into independent-living or assisted-living facilities, nursing homes will be places to care for those who are the most frail and cognitively impaired. Certainly among the services that will be provided (and in most cases, already are provided) are palliative and hospice care, as well as more physical and occupational rehabilitation. In a sense, nursing homes may be transformed into chronic care hospitals.

I have attempted to accurately describe how our system of providing care for the elderly has evolved since our nation began.[22] While the nature of this care and its place in our national culture and psyche has changed, some of the problems – most notably the difficulties

---

21   Many hospitals are converting to private rooms and improving their amenities – for example offering gourmet meals prepared in smaller kitchens, – because today's health care consumers want these changes.

22   Readers in Canada or in other countries with a publicly funded system of health care may take some lessons from the difficulties Americans have encountered in providing this care. The author and editors do not intend to endorse one system of health care over another.

of financing – seem to remain constant. Some of the problems and challenges need a constant and fuller discussion. One of those is how the changes in this industry will impact pastoral care – past, present, or future. The next chapter will explore that in greater detail.

Chapter 24
The Future Of Senior Residential Care:
A Jewish Pastoral Response

Rabbi James Michaels

Scott Janco's previous chapter is eloquent in its setting out the challenges that senior residential care will face in the future. Since he bases his analysis on its history in the United States, I want to add to his remarks by discussing the history of Jewish pastoral care in this area.

As Jewish retirement homes have evolved into centers for specialized care, pastoral care has evolved and taken on a larger role in the overall care programs of these settings. Thirty-five or forty years ago, the average age of residents in such homes was early 70s. Customarily, couples would move into a "retirement home" or "home for the aged" when the bread-winner retired and could no longer afford to own a house; alternatively, individuals would move in when they were widowed and didn't want to live alone or with their children. Mostly comprised of immigrants from Europe, these residents brought their own concepts of Judaism and Jewish observance into their new living environments. Although many were not religious, those who were had the knowledge and ability to conduct religious services, read the Torah, and organize celebrations of religious holidays. When a pastoral need arose, local rabbis would be asked to come to minister to the needs of residents who were their congregants or the parents of their congregants.

In the intervening years, several phenomena occurred. The average age of nursing home residents rose, as people who entered were older and sicker. Those who were healthy retired to warmer climates, or found suitable living accommodations in personal living communities built for seniors. The "type" of Jewish resident also changed. As Americanized children of immigrants, many did not have their parents' knowledge of Jewish practices and observances and thus were no longer able to lead religious services by themselves. Others were prevented from doing this because of physical and/or cognitive disabilities. In addition, in the last decades of the 20th century, administrators of Jewish senior care facilities became more aware of how significant the addition of on-site clinically-trained chaplains (as opposed to an occasional visit from a rabbi) could be to their interdisciplinary teams in working with residents and families. Not only could such personnel take charge of Jewish religious and cultural programs, but they could also add a spiritual dimension set in a psycho-social framework to the care provided by both nurses and social workers.[1]

The Challenges Of The Future

The second decade of the 21st century promises to see many changes to what has become the established model of senior residential care. Several factors will affect this rapid evolution:

Demographic issues: With the first Baby Boomers becoming senior citizens, some will develop conditions and illnesses which will require constant care. Providing this care will be a challenge, regardless of where they choose to receive it. Along with the increased demand for medical care, there will be concomitant spiritual needs and thus a need for pastoral services.

Economic issues: Ironically, even as many Baby Boomers age, some have been thrust into the role of providing care for their own aging parents. Sometimes, this has meant that a two-career couple in which one of the partners retires or loses his/her job has to reevaluate how to provide care for a parent in an independent or assisted living facility. To save on expenses, they may ask the parents to move into their homes, with the unemployed spouse taking on the duties of a caregiver.

Legislated changes: The Affordable Care Act of 2010 contains economic incentives to provide home-based care, making it easier for the elderly to receive care at home. Even though the Obama administration suspended work the CLASS Act, which provided voluntary government-sponsored long-term care insurance, the shift in emphasis to home-based

---

1   Those wishing to learn in depth about the growth of American health care chaplaincy may read Robert Tabak's article, "The Emergence of Jewish Health-Care Chaplaincy: The Professionalization of Spiritual Care" in *American Jewish Archives Journal*, Vol. 62. No. 2, (2010), pp. 89-109.

care will probably be instituted in other ways.

Home-based care: As more people choose their homes as the preferred environment for senior-care, providers of pastoral care will, of necessity, look for new models for providing service. (Indeed, with 80% of seniors today "aging in place", it could be argued that this model is already necessary!) One possible model would resemble that of in-home hospice chaplaincy. In this model, chaplains make scheduled house calls or visit on an as-needed basis. Since it is likely that these chaplains will be dealing with family members as well as with seniors, additional training in family-systems therapy may be advisable.

Another possibility is expanding the concept of the Naturally Occurring Residential Community (NORC). In NORCs, seniors move from larger homes into apartments, which are in buildings and neighborhoods that are conducive to senior living. The example of Florida's Century Village readily comes to mind, but many urban and suburban communities have apartments and condominium communities which attract seniors. Local social service agencies seek out such buildings and focus delivery of service to seniors who live in them. It would be logical to extend pastoral care as an additional service to Jewish NORCs.

In a home-based care environment, providing religious and pastoral services to seniors may be more problematic, as the regularity of chaplaincy visits will be less than those in a senior residential center. One way of addressing this problem is utilizing the technology that is already being used in many skilled nursing facilities. In this case, the Internet would replace closed-circuit television as the means of communication and transmission. While it may be assumed that most baby-boomers using home-care services would be adept in using the Internet, it is also possible that some may have never learned how to use it, or will have lost the ability to "navigate the web." In such circumstances, training caregivers in how to use the Internet most effectively in caring for their loved ones or clients will be necessary. Alternatively, educating seniors in the use of the latest technology could be empowering for them, and also inspiring for their families and caregivers.

Yet another issue that may arise with the growth of home-care will be the sense of dislocation felt by seniors. Specifically, seniors may be moved from their homes in communities they've lived in for many years, and brought to new communities for care but with little opportunity for social interaction. The result may be that they experience significant and prolonged depression. (This phenomenon was observed in 2005 when hundreds of seniors were suddenly transported from New Orleans in the aftermath of Hurricane Katrina.)

One effective pastoral response to this phenomenon might be to provide a "bridge" between their previous homes and their new ones. This would certainly include the chaplains in the seniors' new communities interfacing with rabbis in the seniors' previous communities, especially as they near the end of life. Mobilizing local communities to provide support for families and caregivers will be equally important. Such support might include meals and housekeeping, providing *minyanim* (prayer quorums) and consolation visits during the mourning period of *Shiva*, and follow-up care in the weeks and months thereafter.

Care for younger residents: Although long-term care facilities are usually associated with care for the elderly, many skilled nursing facilities house a number of younger adults. These are usually individuals with physical and/or emotional disabilities who cannot find affordable appropriate care at home. Living among other persons so much older than themselves, they feel an even greater sense of isolation. Disability advocates are currently lobbying Congress to pass the Community Choice Act, which would channel Federal money into locally based care organizations. If this Act becomes law, these individuals will be able to receive care at home, like their older counterparts.

Fran Fulton, executive director of Liberty Resources, a Philadelphia advocacy group for the disabled, says that the Affordable Care Act did include some aspects of the Community Choice Act. However, she says the two biggest issues for the disabled community were not addressed: ending bias in favor of institutionalized care, and the mandate to give people the choice of entering a nursing home or remaining in their own home with community-based services.

Ms. Fulton says the main concern of the younger disabled is isolation. They want access to normal activities at home, at work (if appropriate), and in leisure time activities. She says a proper pastoral way to address the needs of this population would be to focus on providing service for them in individual homes and group settings. Because younger people usually have a greater knowledge of technology, the Internet could be an important means for providing religious services, classes, and individual counseling. In addition, a community-based chaplaincy could work with local congregations and clergy to help empower those who are disabled. This could include advocating for better accessibility in synagogues, special religious services, and more opportunities to integrate the disabled into the larger Jewish community.

Changing roles of institutions: The growth of home-based care does not mean that traditional "brick and mortar" care facilities will no longer be viable. Indeed, they will still be needed by many for whom receiving care at home is no longer a viable option. For example, Alzheimer patients will need the safety of a protected environment to keep them from wandering. Families of patients requiring heavy care may find that a skilled nursing facility is more cost-effective than home-based care; in some situations it may also provide more dignity. Thus, the role of the chaplain will continue to be one which not only facilitates Jewish group activities but also provides individual counseling for residents and family members.

Providing religious services in senior care institutions may pose yet another challenge, as individuals ask for specific services in the style to which they are accustomed (Reform, Reconstructionist, traditional, etc.). As institutions focus more on "person-centered" care, a "one size fits all" Jewish worship service may not suffice; alternative worship choices may be needed, at least on Shabbat and holidays.

The specific needs of Orthodox Jews may need to be accommodated more effectively. For example, if a Jewish facility is not equipped with Shabbat elevators, it may be necessary to create living areas where Orthodox residents can live comfortably so that they do not have to worry about violating Sabbath prohibitions. If such areas for Orthodox residents lack the requisite number of men for a prayer quorum in order to hold worship services (a likely scenario), local congregations may be contacted to help "make a *minyan*" every Shabbat and festival.

New models of care: As Scott Janco states, the model of senior care echoing an acute care setting is rapidly being replaced. As skilled-nursing facilities turn to models of care that are "person-based", chaplains will also have to adapt to these new models by creating and instituting new ways of delivering pastoral care.

One way of adapting is described is described by Sara Pascha-Orlow and Karen Landy in their chapter on the Green House model. In that chapter, they describe opportunities which are available for chaplains in this particular model of long-term care. Almost every aspect of life in the "small houses" they describe – from determining the weekly menu to providing a hands-on method of caring for those at the end of life – entail questions and issues in which Jewish chaplains can be directly involved.

As this particular model of care is instituted in private non-sectarian facilities, a chaplain would still be integral in addressing the needs of Jewish residents in these small communities. Even with a small number of Jewish residents in a community of forty or fifty residents, the chaplain would need to facilitate programs that would not conflict with the facility's overall activities schedule. On the other hand, if the goal of resident empowerment includes sensitizing all residents to the needs of others, then the chaplain's role might include facilitating group discussions about these issues.

In communities where the sole Jewish elder care residence follows the Green House model, different small houses might reflect Jewish religious diversity; residents in the different houses might opt for different modes of religious practice. Thus, a facility with four communities could offer Orthodox, Conservative, Reform and non-observant options. (From a marketing standpoint, such an approach could have tremendous positive implications for generating community support.)

Restaurant-style dining: Over the past few years, I have seen the institution of a new mode of resident dining. At the Hebrew Home of Greater Washington, residents in skilled nursing are served their meals from a steam table on each residential unit, instead of having their individual meals sent on trays from the kitchen. Food is sent in large containers and then is served directly to residents. Because there is always extra food available, a resident who opts for a second helping or a different meal can receive it immediately. The goal is to create an ambience which is more akin to eating in a restaurant.

On Friday evenings and Jewish holidays, a traditional Sabbath or holiday dinner is served with individual *challah* rolls, and small glass goblets of grape juice for *Kiddush* (the blessing inaugurating the sacred day). The program creates a more festive atmosphere. Recorded Jewish music over the public address system also adds to the ambience. Visits by the chaplain, interns, or volunteers can certainly contribute to helping residents celebrate these sacred times.

Responding to staff members: The senior-care industry is highly regulated. With more attention and resources needed to comply with regulations, an increase in stress can be expected among those who work in senior care facilities. And with more stress, there will be a greater need for supportive pastoral care:

– When residents die, the chaplain often conducts memorial services for the deceased and opportunities for loved ones and friends to grieve. When a staff member dies, the chaplain may be in a unique position to provide comfort and pastoral care to the deceased's colleagues and friends in the facilities, especially by conducting a similar service of remembrance.

– As I have written elsewhere in this book, an institution's ethics committee can serve as a central venue for staff to bring concerns regarding the care and treatment of residents.

– The chaplain can provide pastoral counseling for staff unable to consult with their own clergy persons. Because the chaplain is already familiar with the facility and how it runs, staff may feel more comfortable talking with him/her about job-related matters.

– When state and federal surveyors are in the facility, the chaplain can help raise morale. If the survey reveals deficiencies, the chaplain can provide inspiration to staff for performance improvement.

– When local or national tragedies occur, the chaplain can and should organize memorial services, both to respond to the event, and to provide opportunities for the expression of grief.[2]

Conclusion

Over the past decade, senior residential care has undergone rapid and significant changes. Economic, social, and regulatory changes in the coming years will undoubtedly see more challenges and opportunities.

Throughout history, Jews and Jewish communities have always responded to changing social and cultural circumstances. At this point in time, we can see the future of senior care. As the Baby Boom Generation enters its senior years, the need to provide spiritual comfort and guidance for them and their families will continue to grow and evolve. Will we create new pastoral models to fulfill the need? This is the question that we who are concerned about the welfare of Jewish seniors must address. In doing so, may we work to fulfill the Jewish people's mission of bringing *kedushah* / sanctity to the world.

Let us begin.

---

2   Editor's note: In many facilities, such observances were held after 9/11 and are still held on its anniversary – CK.

Contributor Biographies

Kate Brown received a Master of Arts degree in speech-language pathology from The Ohio State University. Her career as a rehabilitation director in skilled nursing facilities has allowed her to focus on the needs of aging adults. She also receives a daily education on flexibility and caring from her twins, Morgan and Jackson, and her husband Matthew.

Susan Buchbinder has been on staff at CJE SeniorLife in Chicago for over 20 years, most recently as Director of Religious Life, providing Jewish cultural competency training for staff and attending to the religious and spiritual needs of CJE's clients. She co-authored an article in the Spring 2008 issue of *Journal on Jewish Aging Services* entitled "Organizational Jewish Values: Honoring the 'J' in CJE SeniorLife." Ms. Buchbinder received her Master's degree from Jane Addams School of Social Work at University of Illinois at Chicago in 1979. She earned a Certificate of Jewish Learning from the Florence Melton Adult Mini-School, a program of Hebrew University, in 2006.

Ellen Cahn received her DHL (Doctor of Hebrew Literature) in Jewish Philosophy from The Jewish Theological Seminary of America; her dissertation was entitled *When Our Strength Fails Us: Jewish Biomedical Considerations about Dementia* which applies Jewish teachings to contemporary ethical problems. An article "Dementia and the Nursing Home Decision" appeared in the Summer 2006 issue of *Conservative Judaism* (58:4,32-50). She is a board certified chaplain with experience in nursing homes and hospitals.

Rabbi Daniel Coleman, BCC, is staff chaplain at North Shore University Hospital (Manhasset, NY), where he is recognized for his community outreach, and compassionate spiritual care to patients, visitors and staff of all faiths as well as non-believers. He has worked in long-term care facilities and various assisted-living facilities in the Bronx. He serves on the Executive Board of the National Association of Jewish Chaplains (NAJC), UJA's Spiritual Care Task Force, and the Bikkur Cholim Coordinating Council's advisory committee. Rabbi Coleman facilitates media programs at North Shore's Center for Extended Care

& Rehabilitation that have been transmitted live to homebound elderly across the U.S.

Paula David, MSW, PhD, teaches full time in the MSW Program at the Factor Inwentash Faculty of Social Work at the University of Toronto. Her research explores the impact of early life trauma on aging with a focus on older adults who are Holocaust survivors. Her interest in the long-term effects of war and genocide grew over the many years she spent at the Baycrest Centre for Geriatric Care developing the Holocaust Resource Program. Her publications include *Caring for Aging Holocaust Survivors – A Practice Manual*, based on her work with survivors and their caregivers.

Deborah Del Signore, M.A.A.T., A.T.R.-BC has a B.A. in Psychology from Hamilton College and a M.A. in Art Therapy from the University of Illinois at Chicago. Deborah has been with CJE SeniorLife since 1999 as a practicing art therapist serving the older adult residents of Lieberman Center, Skokie, IL. She is currently the Manager of Special Programs at Lieberman which encompasses the positions of: Director, Alzheimer's Special Care Unit; Manager, Creative Arts Therapies; and Manager, Life Enrichment Services. Deborah also teaches ethics, assessment and supervision to art therapy graduate students at The School of the Art Institute of Chicago. In April of 2006 she was awarded the Shining Star Award from Life Services Network, an Illinois aging organization. She is the co-creator of the *InnerViews* Film Program which makes documentary films about individuals living in senior residential facilities for the purposes of improving care relationships. Through her work, Deborah explores how ongoing self-expression can improve the lives and communities of older adults living with psychological, cognitive, social and physical challenges.

Linda S. Frank, BSN, CTS, is a commissioned deaconess in the United Methodist Church, serving as the Christian Chaplain for Wexner Heritage Village in Columbus Ohio. Prior to her career change to chaplaincy, she was employed as a Registered Nurse for 30 years working in intensive care, pediatrics, and hospice. She most enjoys spending time with her husband, Doug, her three adult children and their spouses and her grandchildren. She enjoys listening to music in live venues, serving in her home congregation, and relaxing outdoors.

Rabbi David Glicksman, BCC, served as Director of Pastoral Services at the Oscar and Ella Wilf Campus for Senior Living in Somerset, New Jersey from 1991 until 2010. He was born in the Bronx, New York, and received his BA, MS, and Rabbinic Ordination from Yeshiva University. From 1970-1988, he served congregations in Highland Park, NJ and Kansas City, MO. He received board certification from the National Association of Jewish Chaplains and the College of Pastoral Supervision and Psychotherapy. He currently is a Supervisor in Training under the auspices of Robert Wood Johnson University Hospital; his training site is the Center of Hope Hospice in Scotch Plains, NJ. He is married to Leah, a bilingual teacher in the North Plainfield Public School system, and has three children and eleven grandchildren.

Scott Janco is Fellow in the American College of Healthcare Executives and has more than fifteen years experience in health care marketing, strategic planning, and administration. His experience includes community hospitals, medical centers, integrated health care systems, and long-term care organizations. A native of Gary, Indiana, he earned his Bachelor's degree from Indiana University, Bloomington, Indiana and a Master's Degree from Roosevelt University in Chicago. In addition, he has served on Boards of several civic, social services, and not for profit health care organizations.

The Rev. James K. Jensen is an ordained pastor of the Evangelical Lutheran Church in America and a Board Certified Member of the Association of Professional Chaplains. Until his recent retirement from senior residential care chaplaincy, he served as Chaplain at Lutheran Village of Columbus, Columbus, OH for 14 1/2 years and then Summit's Trace and Kensington Place (both in Columbus) for two years.

Rabbi Karen Landy is the staff chaplain at Hebrew Rehabilitation Center at NewBridge on the Charles. In addition she serves as the rabbi for Havurat Shalom, a Reconstructionist congregation in Andover, MA. Karen is a 1997 graduate of the Reconstructionist Rabbinical College. She received her BA from Connecticut College and an MA from Brandeis. She served as the rabbi for Greater Boston's Jewish Family and Children's Services and has taught at Northeastern University and Hebrew College.

Rabbi Gary J. Lavit, BCC, is Director of Pastoral Care at Hebrew Health Care in West Hartford, CT. He received Rabbinic Ordination and a Master's degree in Jewish Philosophy from Yeshiva University, and a Sacred Theology Master's, in Hospital Ministry, from Yale University Divinity School. He is a Board Certified Chaplain of the Association of Professional Chaplains and the National Association of Jewish Chaplains.

Rabbi Beverly W. Magidson has been Director of Chaplaincy Services for the Jewish Federation of Northeastern New York since 1999. She was ordained at the New York School of the Hebrew Union College-Jewish Institute of Religion in 1979 and is a member of the Rabbinical Assembly. This program reaches out to Jews in long-term care facilities throughout the Capital District, particularly those in facilities not under Jewish auspices. She has also been a chaplain at Daughters of Sarah Nursing Center, the Capital District Psychiatric Center, and Albany Medical Center Hospital. She lives in Albany with her husband and is the mother of two grown children.

Naomi Mark, A.C.S.W., is a Licensed Clinical Social Worker in private practice, and currently the Deputy Director of Staff Development at the Human Resources Administration of New York City. Ms. Mark was trained at the Columbia University School of Social Work and at the Ackerman Institute for the Family. She has served as an adjunct clinical professor of social work at Columbia University School of Social Work, a faculty member at the Institute of Psychosocial Oncology and a student educational coordinator at Memorial Sloan Kettering Cancer Center where she also served on its hospital-wide ethics committee. She also served as the book review editor of the academic journal *Social Work Forum.*

Rabbi Sharon Mars is the Jewish Community Chaplain for Greater Columbus. In this role, she attends to members of the Jewish community who are in Columbus' hospitals, nursing homes, correctional facilities, and the Zusman Community Hospice at Wexner Heritage Village. She has also worked in congregations, summer camps, Jewish community centers, and served as campus rabbi for North Carolina Hillel in Chapel Hill for five years. Rabbi Mars is married to Or, and they have three children – Adi, Tova, and Tal.

Leonie Nowitz is the Director of the Center for Lifelong Growth, in New York City, which provides consultation, assessment and care management services to older adults and their families. Ms Nowitz is graduate of Columbia University School of Social Work, and received a Post Master's certificate in Clinical Social Work specializing in Family Therapy. She has taught locally and nationally, and has written extensively on care management issues, working with families and accessing spiritual resources for older people and their caregivers.

Rabbi Sara Paasche-Orlow, BCC, has served since 2003 as the Director of Religious and Chaplaincy Services at Hebrew SeniorLife (HSL) in Boston. In this position she established the HSL Chaplaincy Institute, with a CPE program and pastoral volunteer groups. Sara was ordained at the Jewish Theological Seminary, was a Wexner and then a CLAL fellow, co-founded an American/Israel education program called the Bavli-Yerushalmi Project, and also a non-profit to promote service learning opportunities for Jewish youth and college students. She is married to Dr. Michael Paasche-Orlow and is the mother of three children.

Hedy Peyser, a licensed, certified social worker, serves as Director of Volunteers at the Charles E. Smith Life Communities. She is also the chairperson of its Institutional Review Board and was a Professorial Lecturer in Sociology at The American University. She is responsible for a volunteer corps of over 1,400 and has been recognized for her outstanding contribution to volunteer programming with three AAHSA Outstanding Program Awards, two AJAS awards, including "Mentor of the Year" (2010) and another for outstanding programming. Montgomery County, recognized her work, with the Pyramid Award for professional leadership, and Sulam a local organization assisting individuals with special needs honored her at a dinner. Volunteers serving under her supervision have received state and local recognition, including the "Governor's Award for Outstanding Volunteer Service." She has published numerous articles in professional journals and has also presented papers at national and international conferences. She has served on the Governor's Commission on Volunteerism, and has been featured in the Who's Who Among Human Service Professions, Who's Who of American Women, and the Who's Who in the East.

Dr. Stephen Sapp has taught at the University of Miami since 1980. He is the author of numerous articles on the role of religion, spirituality, and aging and is the author of three books – *Sexuality, the Bible, and Science* (1977); *Full of Years: Aging and the Elderly in the Bible and Today* (1987); and *Light on a Gray Area: American Public Policy on Aging* (1992), and a widely distributed booklet, *When Alzheimer's Disease Strikes* (rev. ed. 2002). Dr. Sapp is past chair of the Governing Council of the Forum on Religion, Spirituality, and Aging (FoRSA) of the American Society on Aging (ASA) and edited FoRSA's newsletter, *Aging & Spirituality*, from 1993 to 1999. He was the 2002 recipient of the ASA Award, the organization's highest award for contributions to the field of gerontology, and the 2010 FoRSA Award. Founding president of the South Florida Chapter of the Alzheimer's Association, from 1990 to 2007 Dr. Sapp chaired the Bioethics Committee of Miami Children's Hospital, where he was Fellow in Clinical Ethics in the Division of Critical Care Medicine in 1996.

Sheila Segal, M.A., B.C.C., until her recent retirement, was Leonard I. Green Chair in Spiritual Care and Director of Chaplaincy Services at the Madlyn and Leonard Abramson Center for Jewish Life in North Wales, PA. After two decades in publishing, including her tenure as Editor-in-Chief of the Jewish Publication Society, Sheila's interest in spiritual life led her to a career in chaplaincy, serving in hospital, hospice, and long-term care settings. She was a co-founder of the Abramson Center's innovative palliative care program and has given numerous presentations on spiritual care at the end of life. Her professional publications include a chapter on "Pain and Suffering" in *Behoref Ha-Yamim: A Liberal Jewish Guide to Decision-Making at the End of Life* (RRC, Center for Judaism and Ethics, 2002). Chaplain Segal is Immediate Past Vice-President of the National Association of Jewish Chaplains.

Joshua Stanton is co-Founder of Lessons of a Lifetime at the Hebrew Home of Greater Washington, Founding co-Editor of the *Journal of Inter-Religious Dialogue* at Auburn Theological Seminary, and co-Director of Religious Freedom USA. He is also a Schusterman Rabbinical Fellow and Weiner Education Fellow at the Hebrew Union College – Jewish Institute of Religion in New York City. A regular writer for the *Huffington Post* and *Tikkun Daily* and member of the Commentators'

Bench at Odyssey Networks, Joshua has had articles and interviews featured in newspapers, radio and television broadcasts, academic journals, and publications in over nine languages. He is also a sought-after speaker, having delivered a keynote address at the 2010 "Eighth Annual Doha Conference," sponsored by the Foreign Ministry of Qatar and the closing address at the November 2009 Tripartite Forum on Interfaith Cooperation at the United Nations.

Index

CPSIA information can be obtained at www.ICGtesting.com
Printed in the USA
BVOW022140080113

310059BV00003B/8/P